Praise from Experts Who Dedicate Their Lives to Women's Health

"Pregnancy after 40 can be a joyful and healthy experience, despite what so many women are led to believe. In her book, *The Joy of Later Motherhood*, Bettina Gordon-Wayne lays out the territory to later motherhood with wisdom and knowledge."

— **CHRISTIANE NORTHRUP**, *MD, OB/GYN,*
and author of New York Times bestsellers: Goddesses
Never Age: The Secret Prescription for Radiance, Vitality,
and Well-Being; Women's Bodies, Women's Wisdom; and
The Wisdom of Menopause

"Bettina Gordon-Wayne has collected powerful and encouraging real-life stories to bring you perspective and resources for your journey to motherhood and to remind you that you are not alone. It's about time the positive science of mature motherhood reached a wider audience."

— **ALISA VITTI**, *functional nutritionist and*
hormone expert, bestselling author of WomanCode,
founder of the FLO Living Hormone Center and creator
of MyFLO app

"I've successfully worked with hundreds of clients worldwide who were 40 and over and got pregnant naturally. I'm thrilled Bettina Gordon-Wayne has collected these powerful stories of women who defied age prejudice and took charge of their own health, fertility, and destiny. The advice shared in this book is invaluable!"

ANDREW LOOSELY, *Chinese medicine*
natural fertility expert, author, and speaker

T0163748

"Women today are not only living longer but we are healthier and have so much to offer a child in terms of life experience and stability. So why shouldn't we have children in our 40s and beyond? I can highly recommend Bettina's book. It is inspiring and empowering. This book will make you think twice about that outdated age paradigm and help you reframe any limiting beliefs."

– CLAUDIA SPAHR, fertility expert, bestselling author, mother of three at 40+, and founder of the popular mother-child yoga retreats Holy-Mama

Praise from Experts Who Thrive to Empower Women

"This book is a *must read* for any woman who wants to start a family after the age of 35. The way this book combines inspiring, real-life stories with data about becoming a mother past the culturally accepted time is so needed. Reading this book is a hope infusion and will be sure to increase your fertility!"

– KATE NORTHRUP, bestselling author of Money: A Love Story and founder of the premier mother-entrepreneur membership site Origin Collective.

"This book will change how you approach motherhood in later life. As a success coach for the past two decades, I've found a need in the market that this phenomenal book now fills—finally, a book I can wholeheartedly recommend to my clients.

"The key element is that Gordon-Wayne focuses on what is possible, rather than dwelling on limitations. She first makes us aware of the massive upsides to motherhood after the age of 40 and then strategically sets out the physical, material, emotional, intellectual, and spiritual options so that the reader can maximize her prospects for having a positive pregnancy experience and a healthy baby."

– JUDYMAY MURPHY, internationally renowned success coach, bestselling author, and speaker

"Becoming a mother is one of the more sacred acts a woman can undertake. Unfortunately, for women over 40, the option is often clouded by fear, inefficient data, and shame. Bettina Gordon-Wayne, through her own story and those of many other women, is taking a stand for natural and healthy pregnancies by creating a new narrative. I imagine you'll feel similarly when you read her extensively researched words of encouragement and hope."

– **MINDIE KNISS**, *entrepreneur, spiritual teacher, and founder of Cor Coaching Academy and HeartPath retreat series*

"While it may be slightly surprising to see a man heaping such high praise on a book written for 'later in life' aspiring moms, I can assure you this terrific book will be a must-read recommendation for many of my female clients worldwide, as the stories and words in the pages of this book absolutely ring true with their most private thoughts, fears, and hopes.

"Bettina Gordon-Wayne has done a masterful job in assembling this book. It has all the research and sourcing of a seasoned journalist, and at the same time, it pulls in readers (yes, even men apparently) as it takes them on a journey that educates, entertains, and empowers women simultaneously."

– **DAVE ELLIOTT**, *international relationship expert, author of The Catch Your Match Formula, founder of Legendary Love For Life*

Praise from Women for Whom This Book Was Written

"Wow—what a great read! These are stories everyone should hear, not just those contemplating starting a family. As an urban professional, almost all my peers are like the women in this book. Bettina does a wonderful job of not just sharing the hope—healthy pregnancies to women of "a certain age" do happen *much* more often than the media tells us—but also sharing the humanity around each of the stories. Brilliant!!"

– **MELANIE**, *45, grant writer*

"Getting to sit and read Bettina's inspiring book tonight with a purring cat beside me was better than going to a spa! The pages are full of energy and life and hope, encapsulated in turns of phrase that make excellent takeaways. For instance, 'mature motherhood' is my new favorite phrase because it replaces all the judgment and fear of being mistaken for a grandma with being an unusually good mother (lucky kid!).

"I also really appreciated the perspective that the '40s are the best decade of a woman's life' and that this is not just an acceptable or possible time to have a baby—but the perfect time to have a child!"

— **ALLISON**, *38, attorney*

"Bettina Gordon-Wayne is the companion that every woman needs on her journey to motherhood. Ebullient and engaging, she offers readers a wellspring of information, insight, and inspiration that are essential to achieving a healthy pregnancy. I know of no other book on the market that does so as effectively. This is a must read for anyone who is struggling with infertility or who is thinking of becoming a mom."

— **RACHEL**, *39, editor*

"In this beautifully written book, the author shares with us, in an engagingly personal voice as if over a shared cup of coffee, her own story of the journey to pregnancy. And then, as if inviting others to the table, she presents her interviews with a wide range of women, who, each on her own unique journey, happened to arrive at motherhood for the first time in her 40s. It's an incredible privilege to read these intimate stories, and to learn how different women responded to the various challenges, upsets, and opportunities on their paths to pregnancy.

"Furthermore, the overall orientation of the author's questions and commentary reveal a reverence and respect for the temples that are our bodies, and a reminder to honor ourselves and our bodies at every stage of life."

— **HANNAH**, *43, environmental expert*

The Joy of Later Motherhood

For Hunter
I am so happy you are here

the Joy *of* Later Motherhood

Your Natural Path to Healthy Babies
EVEN IN YOUR 40s

Bettina Gordon-Wayne

NEW YORK

LONDON • NASHVILLE • MELBOURNE • VANCOUVER

The Joy of Later Motherhood
Your Natural Path to Healthy Babies Even in Your 40s

Published in New York, New York, by Morgan James Publishing. Morgan James is a trademark of Morgan James, LLC. www.MorganJamesPublishing.com

The Morgan James Speakers Group can bring authors to your live event. For more information or to book an event visit The Morgan James Speakers Group at www.TheMorganJamesSpeakersGroup.com.

ISBN 9781683506812 paperback
ISBN 9781683506829 eBook
Library of Congress Control Number: 2017911552

Cover Design by:
Rachel Lopez
www.r2cdesign.com

Interior Design by:
Chris Treccani
www.3dogcreative.net

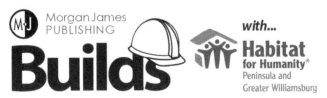

In an effort to support local communities, raise awareness and funds, Morgan James Publishing donates a percentage of all book sales for the life of each book to Habitat for Humanity Peninsula and Greater Williamsburg.

Get involved today! Visit
www.MorganJamesBuilds.com

TABLE OF CONTENTS

Preface I   *Is This Book Right for You?*   xi
Preface II   *Do We Have a Fertility Crisis on Our Hands?*
                   Is It Age Related?   xv
Introduction   *How this Book Started for Me, the Author*   xxvii

Chapter 1   Pillar One: MIND   1
Chapter 2   Let's Honor Our Female Ancestors   15
Chapter 3   Aimee   27
Chapter 4   Leah   35
Chapter 5   Jenny   45
Chapter 6   Ellen   53
Chapter 7   MIND Action Steps   61
Chapter 8   Pillar Two: BODY   67
Chapter 9   Larissa   81
Chapter 10   Darviny and Bernadette   89
Chapter 11   Pippa and Denise   97
Chapter 12   Elise   107
Chapter 13   Claudia S.   115
Chapter 14   BODY Action Steps   123

Chapter 15   Pillar Three: SPIRIT   137
Chapter 16   Claudia C.   151
Chapter 17   Stella   159
Chapter 18   Tamara   167
Chapter 19   Shule Marie   175
Chapter 20   Monique   183
Chapter 21   SPIRIT Action Steps   191

Thank You and Let's Stay in Touch   *205*
About the Author   *209*

PREFACE I

Is This Book Right for You?

In 1970, just 1 percent of first children were born to women over the age of 35. In 2012, this number shot up to 15 percent in the United States and was even higher in some European countries. In 2016, while the birthrate among women under the age of 30 was at an historical low in America, the birthrate for women ages 40 to 44 was up 4 percent from the previous year. Celebrities like Salma Hayek, Halle Berry, Gwen Stefani, Tina Fey, and Eva Mendez all rocked their glamorous baby bumps beyond their big 4-0. For every mature mom-to-be who wonders if she'll be the only one on the playground with graying hair and laugh lines, this is wonderful and encouraging news. Welcome to later motherhood!

Now, brace for impact.

A quick Google search for advice and inspiration on "pregnancy over 35" will hit a hopeful mother-to-be right in the gut. She'll find over forty-eight million websites, the vast majority containing negative headlines and anxiety-inducing statistics about increased physical, mental, and whatever-else risks for mother and child. A Google search of "pregnancy over 40" will make her want to declare herself insane for even thinking she could have a healthy, naturally conceived child at her age—unless, of course, she is willing to buy into the four-billion-dollar-a-year infertility business and drain her bank account on costly treatments.

I respectfully and wholeheartedly disagree with this point of view.

My name is Bettina Gordon-Wayne, and I am the third generation of women in my family who did not get the memo that motherhood in our 40s is dangerous, if not outright impossible. My grandmother had her second child at 42. My mother had me at 42. And I got easily and naturally pregnant at 43, the very first time my husband and I tried in earnest to conceive (after a big fail two years earlier). I delivered our healthy son through a natural and unmedicated birth at age 44. A couple of years later, I write this book while contemplating a second child.

I've always approached the topic of later motherhood from a position of strength and power, and I strongly feel in my heart that it is time to change the narrative from a doom and gloom scenario to one of hope and possibilities.

Over the course of the last three years, I have used my twenty-plus years of experience as an international journalist to study and research the topic of later motherhood here in the United States and in Europe. And I've uncovered a surprising reality that lies beneath the discouraging statistics and costly infertility treatments: there are a lot more women over 40 (not to mention in their mid and late 30s) who are able to naturally conceive healthy babies than we are led to believe. Some of us 40+ moms conceived our babies with ease, while others overcame adversity, dove deep into self-healing, or methodically got themselves ready for motherhood with the help of natural fertility specialists.

Why don't we know about the success stories? Because our stories are usually not told. *Until now.*

I've interviewed dozens of women who have had one, two, and even three healthy babies after their big 4-0, and I've prepared their stories for you, the reader, in the hope that they will bring you inspiration, guidance, and maybe some solace for the heartaches you may have already faced.

Whatever your experience or concern, chances are, we—the women I interviewed and myself personally—have been there as well. Each and every mother who said yes to sharing such a profound sliver of her life so openly in this book did it out of love and compassion for you, the woman and mother-to-be who opens these pages. We believe in helping each other, and we believe in the eternal female bond that connects us, particularly around the topic of children, birth, and our place in the continuum of the world.

This book contains our stories, our honesty, our tears, our triumphs, our collective wisdom, our advice, our compassion, and, most important, our deep love for all the other women out there who are where we once were: ready to start a family and wondering how it will all pan out.

This book is for you if the following rings true:

- You'd like to approach the topic of mature motherhood from a position of strength and power.
- You have a hunch that there is more to conceiving a child than just the physical act, and you are curious as to the experience of others.
- You would like to get pregnant in the near future or in the next couple of years, and you are already worried because of your age.
- You've tried to conceive naturally, but it has not worked out yet. Now, you want input from other women on improving your chances, through physical, mental, and spiritual health.
- You are afraid that your body may fail you. Or that your contradictory thoughts—"I would love to have a baby, but I don't think I can give up my freedom!"—may influence your fertility.
- You feel alone and isolated because you've already experienced more than your fair share of heartache. You need different perspectives to help you go on.
- You're worried you'd be mistaken for "grandma" at the playground and younger parents and society might judge you for your choice.
- You wonder if it is fair to a child to have older parents and whether he'll have to shoulder the burden of an ailing mother or father long before his peers.

You are worried. You are upset. You doubt that motherhood will ever happen for you. We get it. We've been there. At least one of us has your back, maybe more. With our stories, we want to lovingly see you through this journey as much as we can.

We've got you.

Do We Have a Fertility Crisis on Our Hands? Is It Age Related?

Before we dive deep into all the positive aspects of mature motherhood, let's talk about the big white elephant in the room: Why does it seem like we have a fertility crisis on our hands? And is it all related to age?

(FYI: this is one of the rare spaces in the book where you will read the word "infertility," as this is one of the most damaging words to a woman's psyche when she's in the vulnerable space of opening up to new life.)

Regardless of how old you are, let me ask you a question: How many women and men do you personally know or at least know of who had trouble conceiving? How many of your friends used assisted reproductive technology (ART) to get pregnant? Are you yourself one of them?

We all personally know or know of a couple who had difficulties conceiving and were labeled infertile. Infertility is defined as not being able to get pregnant after one year of trying or after six months if a woman is 35 years of age or older. Women who can get pregnant but are unable to stay pregnant may also be considered infertile. According to the Centers for Disease Control and Prevention (CDC), about 12 percent of women (seven million) in the United States, aged 15–44 years, have difficulty getting pregnant or staying pregnant because their own fertility or that of their partner is compromised.

In their 2015 report, *Infertility in America* (isn't that a cold, ugly title?), the Reproductive Medicine Associates of New Jersey state that there has been a 65 percent increase in in vitro fertilization (IVF) since 2003.

Today it seems almost naïve to think that baby-making is just a question of well-timed sex. And it's not just couples of a "certain age"—even couples as young as their 20s and early 30s report having problems conceiving a healthy child and carrying the baby to term. It's the truth: infertility is on the rise. But why is that?

If you read media reports, many online blogs, and fertility clinic publications— and believe me, I have—you will find one thread throughout: for women, age remains the single-most significant factor impacting fertility. Fertility drops at 35 and goes into free fall after 40. If a woman experiences infertility, it's because she waited too long. It's because she did not make motherhood her priority. It's because she pursued higher education and focused on her career. And now her eggs are too old. It's her fault and hers alone.

Really?

I am not writing this book to regurgitate what you can easily find elsewhere. I am writing this book to add new perspectives to the topic and to add new voices from women whose experiences have borne out that having healthy babies past your 40th birthday may be more common and natural than we are led to believe. It may not be without struggle, but it's certainly not uncommon.

I am also sharing here the clinical results of holistic health practitioners who treated some of these women and whose work has a higher success rate than high-tech fertility clinics (in vitro fertilization statistically only works successfully as little as 20-21 percent of the time for women in their late 30s and possibly only 10–11 percent of the time for women over 40. FYI: Almost one in five pregnancies through assisted reproductive technology [ART] do not result in a live birth. The success rate is calculated on live births).

So here is the big nugget: In my extensive research into the topic of fertility, I have come to understand that fertility is an extension of our health—not just our physical health but also our emotional, mental, and spiritual health. I've learned that we should not look at fertility as being something singular that may or may not go haywire within our bodies at a certain age, but rather see fertility as one piece in the puzzle of our body's intricate web of life. And this elaborate web of health and wellness includes what we think, what we feel, and the stories we tell ourselves.

Age Is *Not* the Biggest Deciding Factor; Overall Health Is

If our mental, emotional, and physical health is well tended to and our organs and sensitive biological systems, like the endocrine (hormonal) or immune system, work optimally, a woman's fertility fires on all cylinders—regardless of her age—as long as she is still menstruating and ovulating regularly. But if we don't take optimal care of our bodies and minds—I, for one, don't know a single person who consistently does that for years—the system gets compromised, whether we are aware of it or not.

Chances are, we may overlook the symptoms. We might think that the bloated belly is because of the slice of pizza, not because of chronic inflammation in our gut. We forget that we have hormonal imbalances because we have long suppressed any symptoms by taking the pill. We shrug off lower back pain as due to an uncomfortable mattress instead of recognizing the deterioration of our musculoskeletal system from sitting in front of a screen all day. Or we deny that we are emotionally sickened from the pressure we are under at work and keep ourselves running on coffee and numbed on sweets and alcohol.

We may look—and still be—young and vibrant on the outside, yet our inner system may be breaking down like a house of cards the minute one too many cards is removed. When reality hits, it may show up in an area of our lives we hold dear: the opportunity to give and bring new life into the world.

So, in order to understand what is going on, we need to look at something so intimate and sacred as conceiving and bearing life and put this miracle—and it is nothing short of that—into the larger context of living at the beginning of the third millennium.

All the interviews I conducted and the research I did led me to this conclusion: a lack of fertility is the manifestation of the lifestyle we lead and the environmental toxins we absorb in the twenty-first century.

Here is the reality of why today's women and men in their fertile years run into more challenges than previous generations did:

- As a society at large, we have become rather ill. According to the CDC, about half of all adults—117 million people—has one or more chronic health conditions. One out of four adults has two or more chronic health conditions.

- Autoimmune diseases are on the rise and are three times more likely to afflict women, most of them in their childbearing years, than men. According to the American Autoimmune Related Diseases Association, there are fifty-plus million Americans who are struggling with numerous autoimmunity issues, such as multiple sclerosis, rheumatoid arthritis, inflammatory bowel disease, fibromyalgia, Hashimoto's thyroiditis, etc.

- Our hormones are out of whack. Millions of American women don't ovulate regularly—or at all. 5–10 percent of women of childbearing age are affected by polycystic ovarian syndrome (PCOS). According to the PCOS Foundation, PCOS is responsible for 70 percent of infertility issues in women who have difficulty ovulating. Primary ovarian insufficiency (POI) is another cause of ovulation problems. POI and PCOS are both clear indicators that a woman's hormonal balance is compromised.

- We eat too many unhealthy foods. According to the CDC, more than two thirds of Americans are overweight; 38 percent are even obese. Between the early 1970s and 2010, the obesity rate more than doubled. In other words, over seventy-eight million US adults and about 12.5 million (16.9 percent) children and adolescents are obese—not just overweight, obese.

- Nearly one in four women, 23.4 percent, are obese before becoming pregnant, which can increase the risk of a wide range of health complications for the baby and the mother. More than 6 percent (approximately one in sixteen) of pregnant women have or develop diabetes during pregnancy—known as gestational diabetes.

- Our food supply consists of vegetables sprayed with pesticides, antibiotic- and growth-hormone-injected meat, and packaged foods that are void of nutrients, yet can include ingredients that are banned in other countries because of their risk to consumers' health. Personally, I am appalled by every company that sells a healthier version of their product—household staples like mac and cheese—in Europe, while still keeping the ingredients that are labeled unsafe in other countries in their American products. Check out *foodrevolution.org* or *foodbabe.com* for facts.

- We don't move. 80 percent of American adults do not meet the government's national physical activity recommendations for aerobic exercise and muscle strengthening.

- We are glued to our screens. In the United States, people spend an average of 444 minutes every day looking at screens, or 7.4 hours. That breaks down to 147 minutes spent watching TV, 103 minutes in front of a computer, 151 minutes on a smartphone, and 43 minutes with a tablet.

- We are nature and sunlight deprived. According to the Environmental Protection Agency, the average American spends 93 percent of his life indoors, 6 percent of which is spent driving. That means we are outdoors for only 7 percent of our lives, equivalent to one half of one day per week.

- We are constantly exposed to endocrine (hormone) disruptors in our environment. If you wash your hair often and use conventional brand conditioner or hair styling products or if you apply makeup on a regular basis or use body lotions and sunscreens, you've been building up toxins in your body for years and years. The same goes for household cleaning products, the chemicals in air fresheners or, for example, nail polish. If a product is for sale at a US supermarket, drugstore, or department store cosmetics counter, it does *not* mean it is safe to use (check out *http://www.ewg.org/skindeep/myths-on-cosmetics-safety/*).

- Depending on what statistics you look at, the rate of how miserable most Americans feel at work is alarming: between 53 percent and 70 percent of those surveyed in the last couple of years hate their jobs or are completely disengaged—not even incentives and extras can excite them. As a woman, you can bet that pressure at work, high stress levels, and any overall unhappiness will take its toll on your body and soul.

- Women and girls are victims of violence. One in four women in the United States will experience domestic violence at some point in their lives. Trauma, like assault, rape, miscarriage, abortion, and even adoption, can have a significant impact on a woman's ability to conceive, as I learned in many interviews with holistic fertility specialists. Many times, the victim thinks that she has overcome her trauma already, only to realize that more work needs to be done before she can give life to the next generation.

This is our reality in America, but the rest of the Western world is not much better off. And we have not even touched the mental and emotional factors that can have a profound influence on fertility as well.

Somehow, fertility issues are seen as a woman's problem. In reality, infertility affects women and men alike, but usually we women get blamed for having waited too long—thus having squandered our fertility. The fact is, for one third of infertility cases, it is the man's sperm that is not viable; for one third of cases, both the woman and the man are challenged; and for one third of cases, it's the woman's fertility that is compromised—regardless of age.

Having said all of this, here is the great news: fertility is changeable and can improve when we start to see it as part of the bigger system, as part of our overall health.

Could it be more difficult for couples over 35 and over 40 to conceive? Yes. Is it primarily because of the woman's age? You now have enough information to decide that for yourself. Can you improve your fertility and your chances? Yes!

But What about Health Risks to the Baby?

Do certain risks increase with age? Yes. I am not trying to downplay the risks of improper chromosome division—the probability of Down syndrome, for example, increases with age. The majority of these pregnancies will miscarry naturally.

It is a very sad truth that, among women in their childbearing years who know they are pregnant, ten to twenty-five out of every one hundred will experience a miscarriage. That doesn't even take into account the 50–75 percent of all fertilized eggs that are aborted spontaneously, usually before the woman even knows she is pregnant.

My own mother had eight (!) miscarriages between the age of 23 and 40. I am child number ten, the second one that survived, the only girl, and the last of my mother's pregnancies, at age 42. (My mother is a biochemist. Back in the fifties and sixties, the doctors did not make the connection between dangerous chemical fumes in the laboratory and dying fetuses).

Two of my closest friends, one at 31, the other at 39, chose to abort rather than birth a severely handicapped child into the world. Another dear friend recently found out that her two-year-old girl has a genetic disorder that delays her development and will influence the rest of her life. The girl's condition did not show up in the genetic testing during pregnancy. In fact, the condition is so rare, it does not even have a name yet. Her mother now lays awake at night wondering if her precious girl will ever attend school, find somebody to love, or be able to live on her own one day. Even though the doctors said that her genetic mutation was not related to her parents' age, the girl's mom, my friend, wonders if being over 40 when she naturally conceived may still have had an influence.

The truth is, creating life, whether naturally or aided by medical technology, can be heartbreaking and full of challenges and risks. This book cannot take the risks away, nor can it promise you a baby, but it can offer you a new perspective on pregnancy and motherhood.

You will read about women who overcame the very health challenges I mentioned earlier or who mastered their mindset to still hold out for their naturally conceived child, even after multiple miscarriages. This book will show you what is possible and how you can maximize your chances to conceive a healthy and vibrant child naturally after the age of 40.

Do I Recommend That You Should Delay Starting Your Family?

One hallmark of qualitative journalism, my profession since 1992, is that a journalist remains unbiased, preventing her own opinion from influencing her reporting. Having said that, this book is more to me than a news story—it is my personal mission to bring the voices of us 40+ moms to you in the hope of empowering you and taking some of the fear and anxiety out of your journey to motherhood. So, you should know where I personally stand on two particular topics: timing and technology.

The "Best" Time To Have a Baby

Because I am so passionate about and see so many upsides to later motherhood, people often assume that I am encouraging women to delay starting their families. I don't tell any woman who feels ready for her child to wait because what if she runs into trouble conceiving later on? It would be irresponsible of me. What I do say, though, is this: if you are in a loving relationship with a mature partner and you two have weathered stormy times and have emerged stronger for it, why wait? The perfect time for having children may never come because life is always busy and there are always other things to consider. If you are both committed and know you're heading toward starting your family, do it now—if for no other reason than, if you do delay and subsequently experience fertility challenges, you may blame yourself for having waited too long.

But I would never ever encourage a woman who personally does not feel ready yet—is in a stressful financial place or has not found the partner she loves and could depend on to share the responsibility of raising a child—to get pregnant because statistics and fertility doctors recommend that a woman should become a mother by 30, before her fertility declines.

What's the real message here when we pressure women to hurry? Abandon your professional calling and get in line with what society expects from you?

Go and marry the wrong man so that at least you can procreate now? Or have a child out of wedlock—never mind if you are emotionally ready, financially stable, and enthusiastic about raising a human being into adulthood? I think it is irresponsible to tell a woman to bring a new life into this world (and care for this life with all the love and dedication this child deserves for two decades to come) based solely on the age listed on her driver's license.

Personally, I experienced the perfect time for me to have a baby. It was at age 44. I am very sure that I would not have been as happy and content with my new role as a mother if I had my boy at 41—*before* I had worked out my internal struggle (see the Introduction, "How This Book Started for Me, the Author"). Working out my stuff allowed me to become a woman who deeply enjoys being a mother, and thus, I show up for my child with more maturity and grace. Every woman has her own unique and personal timeline when she and her partner are eager to have a child. For some, this is sooner; for others, later.

Assisted Reproductive Technology

I'd also like to tell you, up front, where I stand in regards to assisted reproductive technology (ART), since this book focuses on natural conception only.

As a woman, I am in awe of reproductive science and what we can do today to help women and men have babies. I congratulate every single woman who went through the often arduous and heartbreaking process of ART to become a mother, and I admire her strength and courage.

There are five million human beings in this world who would not be alive if not for reproductive technology, and I personally know many children who were born after their parents sought help at a fertility clinic. For many couples, ART is a blessing and a miracle. The last thing I would want any woman to think is that I, or the other women in this book, would pass judgment on her and her choices of how to bring life to this planet. We are mature women. We are mothers. We support each other's choices.

In fact, quite a few of the women in this book explored their options with fertility clinics and their doctors. That's why I am aware that the infertility services market, from infertility clinics and sperm banks to fertility drugs and surrogacy programs, has become a big business—to the tune of almost four-billion dollars each year, up fourfold from twenty-five years ago. And that not every fertility specialist, no matter how reputable he may be, takes the time to look at a woman in all her complexity, instead of just analyzing her uterus, egg count, and age (to oversimplify it). For some of the women I spoke to, this narrow focus led to considerable frustration and pain.

Rita went to one of the top fertility clinics in New York City and spent well over one-hundred-thousand dollars (money she did not readily have). Sadly, she lost all three of her pregnancies. When her fertility specialist pushed her toward using donor eggs, another costly process, she became disheartened. Neither the fertility doctor, nor her OB/GYN, ever bothered to look for the underlying cause of her miscarriages—it was all blamed on her age of 38 and her "old eggs." But Rita felt in her gut that something was not right with this assessment.

That's when Rita took back her power and, with the help of her sister, a gynecologist, started her own research on what could be going on with her body. Rita also connected with fertility specialist Aimee Raupp (read her story in chapter 3), and Aimee helped diagnose Rita's autoimmune disease and offered guidance on how to heal from it. Today, at age 40, Rita is the mother of a naturally conceived son, and she and Aimee are working together again to prime her for her second pregnancy.

Elise was 45 when she went to a highly regarded fertility clinic in my husband's home town of Chicago. She went there to assess her body's health and to get blood work done to establish her chances of conceiving a biological child. Elise had hardly sat down when the female doctor whipped out a chart and presented to the very surprised Elise the risks of birth defects related to a woman's age.

This doctor could have been talking to the healthiest and most fertile 45-year-old she'd ever met in her life, but she wouldn't have known it as she immediately led the conversation with frightening statistics and anxiety, before seamlessly proceeding to talk about the different procedures the clinic could offer Elise and the payment plans she could choose from. Elise was told that, at her age, she needed to look for an egg donor right away. "Luckily," the clinic offered twenty-four-hour access to their donor list for free, so Elise could peruse it before signing the contract (read Elise's story in chapter 12).

These are just two examples of when the laser focus of surely well-meaning and highly trained fertility specialists completely missed the mark and would have cost both women the biological, naturally conceived children they have today.

In conclusion, let me say this: I hope you find enough value and information in this book that the infertility service market becomes one option, *just not the only one.*

How this Book Started for Me, the Author

(Or, in other words, "Well, Bettina, good for you that you got pregnant on the first try at 43. You really got f***ing lucky!")

Early last year, I reached out to my media colleague Sophie to pitch her my book idea. Sure, I'd been a well-respected journalist myself for over two decades, and I knew a good story when I saw one, but I still needed another perspective as to whether my book idea was, indeed, valid or not. As a top TV producer, Sophie had been pitched to thousands of times before and had developed an uncanny knack for spotting potential winners. I also thought that Sophie, a 44-year-old single woman living in Los Angeles, would be my target audience, as I knew she had deeply longed for a child for years and was exploring her options. She seemed my perfect pitching partner. She became more than that.

"So, tell me your own story," Sophie said and then fell silent on the other end of the phone line.

I was caught off guard. I had prepared a short pitch but, because she'd asked, I shared my story in detail. I told her about Joshua and I getting married when he was in his mid-30s and I was in my late 30s, and how, for years, I was not even sure I wanted to become a mother. Sure, I felt pressure from my environment and our culture to reproduce and do what we women are "born to do," but I wasn't convinced that motherhood was the right path for me. I mean, really, do we women *need* to become mothers just because we can? I don't think so!

At some point, though, I gave in. I had just turned 40, and I had a husband who wanted children—I was not adverse enough for a firm, "No, thank you." I was willing to give it a try. Joshua and I ditched the contraceptives and went for it. And while, outwardly, I said, "Yes, we want children," inwardly, I struggled.

Actually, I was riddled with fear about what the responsibilities of creating and raising a human being would do to my life. I doubted that I could raise a child in America while taking care of my ailing mother in Austria. I struggled because I worried about the idea of putting my child into daycare (growing up, I had been taught that children needed their mommies for the first years of their lives and "good" mothers stayed home with their babies). And yet, I had been working from home for over a decade and longed to get outside the house again. I was deeply lonely and yearned for a team of smart people I could work with and learn from. Try getting that from an infant or a toddler. "A child would be a prison sentence!" was actually one of the thoughts I had. (That's how awful my self-talk was.)

Yet, my biggest fear was the uncertainty of how—or even if—I could handle giving up my hard-earned freedom for the needs of a baby. I was the woman who got stir-crazy after three weeks at home and who needed to travel at least once a month in order to keep my sanity. I had chosen journalism as my profession because of the diversity it brought in terms of topics to cover and fascinating people to meet. If I could neither travel nor report on a whim, but be stuck in the house with an infant, what kind of life would that be? And this one was a biggie as well—what if my relationship with Joshua was not strong enough to withstand the stressors and difficulties of raising a kid? Would I end up a single mother? Would I be stressed, financially broke, and all alone with my child? Oh, my goodness, no, no, *no*!

It turned out, I was anxious about nothing.

All of 2010 came and went, and I did not get pregnant. Nope, nada, not happening. If Joshua and I had gone to a fertility expert at this point, we would have been scolded for having waited so long. And we would have been diagnosed with "unexplained infertility," a label smacked onto about a third of the healthy couples who try to conceive without success.

Right after New Year's 2011, Joshua wanted to get more serious about our baby-making and suggested we should start charting to enhance our chances, and that we should have sex more often during my fertile time. "He became a man on a mission, totally focused on getting me pregnant," I told Sophie. "Two days later, I woke up with severe cramps in my lower abdomen. The pain was so crippling, I couldn't stand upright or walk. It was pain like I had never experienced before."

"What happened?" Sophie asked.

"It was my body telling me why it had not conceived for over a year." Even though I had said that I had wanted kids, I honestly, secretly, and painfully did *not* want them, not really. Eventually my body physically manifested the doubts I had and told me to stop, to stop trying to conceive and to face what was so hard to admit: the risk of completely losing the life I had worked so hard to build was too big for me to take. I cherished my freedom, and I felt duty-bound to my ailing mother in Europe who needed *me* in emergencies, not my brother. I did not want to potentially sacrifice it all for parenthood.

My infertility was the result of my truth—and of my focus on the limitations a child would bring to me, its mother. I realized I had to voice that truth the way my body had spoken to me: in no uncertain terms. On a snowy, gloomy evening in February, I sat my husband Joshua down to tell him that I was sorry, but that I did not want to have children. Not now, maybe never. Then I waited for him to leave me.

It took months for Joshua to decide what had to give: his wish for a child or our marriage. Slowly and deliberately, he came around to accepting that he might never be a father, but that his life would still be rich with love, experiences, and professional success. And it included me, his wife! He made peace with letting go of fatherhood and embraced a life designed according to his work and passions. But as Joshua found his peace, I realized, much to my surprise and utter dismay, that although the whole baby question may have been over for him, it wasn't for *me*!

Silently, in partnership with only myself, I wrestled with many questions: "Is this decision a mistake? Will I regret this in ten years when it's too late? If I had not put my mother's needs—a daughter across the Atlantic who could drop everything on a dime to come to her hospital bed—before mine, would I have decided otherwise?"

I told Sophie about the year that three things happened: I started a brand-new career; Joshua and I went to couples therapy to smooth out some rather rough edges; and we adopted a dog from a high-kill shelter—all of which set the stage for me to change my mind about motherhood and open up my life and body to the spirit of a child. I described to Sophie how I started to look for ways in which a child could enrich my life instead of only filtering for the limitations and sacrifices. I told her how Joshua confided that he would still be open to the idea of starting a family. And how one article that I read in the *Huffington Post* pushed me over the edge and made me firmly stand in my new truth: I did want to become a mother after all. Two years after my initial decision, at age 43, I had totally reversed my mind and changed my heart!

Sophie hadn't said anything for some time, so I continued with enthusiasm: "I read this story on February 22nd, and I instantly lost all my fear. I made the firm decision to choose personal growth over freedom. And I knew that motherhood was right for me and that I would pursue this path."

The next three months, Joshua and I physically and mentally prepared for parenthood. We did multiple things to ready our bodies, like doing a gentle cleanse and eating a very healthy diet, but I believe it was my mindset and deep change of heart, more than anything, that opened my body up for conception. I had no doubt anymore that this was right. In June, when I was 43 and Joshua was 42, we became pregnant the first month we tried.

I was in Italy finishing up my education as a mental strength trainer when I found out that our lives would be forever changed. I took the pregnancy test in a little hut on top of a mountain in the Italian Alps and told Joshua ten days later when we reunited in the harbor of the medieval town of Dubrovnik on the Croatian coast just as the sun was setting. It literally took him minutes to fully realize what I had just told him. We were elated when we heard the baby's heartbeat for the first time. "And guess what the baby's due date was?" I asked Sophie, with my voice raised in excitement. I waited a second for effect: "It was February 22nd, one year to the date of me reading the *Huffington Post* article that changed everything!"

Silence on the other end of the phone. Then a short cough. "That's a nice story," Sophie eventually said.

I could hear in her voice that my experience of ease stirred something up in her and that she was choosing her words carefully now. "But, honestly, there are so many women out there that are really struggling with becoming pregnant in their 40s. I know that, because I read up on it all the time. It is such a loaded topic, full of guilt for having waited too long or shame for bodies that are not working as they should or marriages breaking apart because of the stresses of IVF treatments, not to mention when you try to do it alone. I mean, if you're over 44, most fertility specialists won't even let you try using your own eggs anymore, for Christ's sake!" My heart sank when I heard her pain. I had not meant to hurt her.

"For some women, your story may be inspiring. Others who don't have it that easy may say, 'Well, Bettina, good for you that you got pregnant on the first try at 43. You really got f***ing lucky!'"

Sucker punch.

For days after, I contemplated this sentence. Was I, indeed, just freaking lucky? Or are we, as a society, so focused on struggle and pain and negative statistics that we brush positive news aside as flukes? Sure, I am lucky and very grateful for a textbook pregnancy, a natural, unmedicated birth at 44 and a healthy and strong son who blossoms and develops beyond expectations. I do not take any of it for granted.

Yet, was it all just luck? Maybe. *But what if it wasn't?*

Every time I sat with this question in silence, my gut, my soul, my inner voice would say, "This was not just luck. Don't disregard your experience because it was easy, joyful, and utterly positive."

And I pondered how, over the course of two years, I had turned my infertility into a fertile mindset and a fertile body, ready to conceive and host a baby: "What if I am not the only one with conflicting thoughts that may keep some of us from conceiving, as had happened to me? What if conception is not only a physical event, but an occurrence that is strongly influenced by what we think, feel, and believe? What if Joshua and I did something right to easily conceive and carry our child to term that could help others? Wouldn't that be worth sharing?"

My gut, heart, and soul said *yes*. And then the voice inside me added her professional two cents: "And while you are at it, make use of your twenty-five years in journalism and find other success stories to tell as well."

It was this one conversation with Sophie that changed the course of the book I originally set out to write. Initially, this was a book on motherhood in your 40s, for which I had also interviewed moms who used a variety of ART methods, moms who adopted, and moms who used surrogacy to have their children (these stories will be published in a second book, as they are equally amazing in their unique ways). But it was my phone call with Sophie that made me realize that this book you are holding in your hands needed to be on natural conception and the prevalent myth of "Oh, you conceived naturally later in life? What a fluke!"

So, I set out to find the other moms, the women who conceived naturally and bore healthy children after the age of 40, and guess what? I found many more women with positive and encouraging stories than I ever dreamt of.

I never had to post on my social networks or go to chat groups or engage on fertility sites to find my ladies. Instead, I found them all within my existing circles of friends and acquaintances, or I had friends introduce me to friends of theirs. In half a dozen cases, I even "magnetized" them to me in funny ways. I met Elise while we were both shopping at the supermarket—we bonded in the produce aisle, discussing healthy food choices for our toddlers. I met Shari at the coffee shop next to the White House where I sat to work on the book. Ricky and I met at my neighborhood dog park; Cass and I ran into each other (well, our toddlers did, quite literally) at the National Arboretum, and Jo and I met at the yoga studio where we struck up a pose and conversation and "coincidentally" realized we both fell pregnant past the big 4-0 birthday.

Twice I happened to spot a woman at a friend's party who I figured could maybe be a mature mom (judging the right age is so difficult these days, as we look so much younger than previous generations did), and I would direct the conversation toward that topic. As soon as I enlisted an, "Oh, yes, I had my child in my 40s, too," I would immediately follow up with the most logical question to ask a complete stranger: "Naturally conceived or IVF?"

It was as if the universe was bringing them to me and vice versa. And in my interviews with about sixty of these 40+ moms for this book alone (and many more ever since) and my talks with many holistic health fertility specialists, I made some surprising discoveries.

In our Western world, we tend to think that pregnancy is the result of a physical event and nothing but a physical event, and so we focus on the body, examine it, prod it, and (attempt to) fix it. But after digging deep into this topic and after looking at dozens and dozens of first-person-accounts, I can say with absolute certainty: your mental and emotional well-being and your spiritual beliefs—what meaning you give your life—are the precursors to every single pregnancy. They are the foundation, the bedrock, the underpinning. You can push your body and attempt to fix it all you want, but if you miss these other aspects of fertility, you will not be optimally set up to succeed.

And why wouldn't you want to succeed? We all want you to, so that's why I approach pregnancy and motherhood from three different angles: the mind, the body, and the spirit. These are all aspects in your life that you will need to address in order to maximize your chances for conception.

- The first pillar is dedicated to the MIND, as this seems especially relevant for us older moms who are bombarded with negative messages and age-related worries. Your mind can either hinder your body or support it. You will read stories of women whose mindset was the most conducive for conception (my mother's) and the most problematic (Jenny's).

- The second pillar focuses on the BODY, which is not only your temple but your future baby's home. Our bodies need to be nurtured and well attended to long before conception, like the soil in a garden needs to be tended to before planting seeds. You'll read about women who intentionally healed and primed their bodies for pregnancy and the stunning story of one woman whose body self-healed after an adoption.
- The third pillar, SPIRIT, is really about faith. Whether it's faith in God, spirit, and/or the universe, it's about trusting in divine timing and relinquishing control in order to receive the miracle. Women shared how their faith helped them deal with miscarriages or how they connected to their children before they were even born. If you read closely, though, you will find aspects of each pillar in practically every story.

In addition, I've created an online portal into "Fertility and Health" exclusively for you, the readers of *The Joy of Later Motherhood*. Please go to *BettinaGordon.com/Bonus,* where I published additional interviews with fertility experts and share more advice on how to increase your health and fertility (this information is equally valid and important for women who choose ART). You can also browse photos of the moms featured in the book, enjoy additional bonuses, and be part of our robust and growing community. For everybody who bought one or more copies of this book, access to the interviews and additional information is offered for free as my personal thank you. Since I gathered so much more wisdom, advice, and surprising perspective through my interviews than I could fit into just one book, I created a companion guide called *Sisterhood,* which you will also find in the book bonus section. If you want to reach out to me personally, please drop me a line at *BettinaBook@BettinaGordon.com.*

Hop on over to the website *BettinaGordon.com/Bonus* and join our community so we can all support you on your journey to motherhood and beyond.

With love,

Bettina

CHAPTER 1

Pillar One: MIND

Your Mind Is Stronger Than Your Genes

A couple of years ago, in the dead of winter, I flew to Portland, Maine, and drove in my rental car to the small village of Yarmouth to interview a woman I've deeply respected ever since I read her bestseller, *Women's Bodies, Women's Wisdom*, a book that, frankly, should be in every woman's library. Oprah Winfrey and millions of other women around the world breathed a sigh of relief when Dr. Christiane Northrup put unique female physical challenges—things like cysts, fibroids, and menopause—into the context of a woman's environment, ancestry, thoughts, beliefs, and emotions.

While the majority of the medical establishment was still treating ailments with medication or surgery alone, Dr. Northrup, a board-certified OB/GYN, looked at her patients as complex human beings and recognized the deeper emotional patterns that were expressing themselves physically. It took guts, perseverance, and tenacity to first publish *Women's Bodies, Women's Wisdom* in 1994 (she told me even her own editor on the book pushed back), but today, Dr. Northrup is undeniably one of the world's leading voices in "all that can go *right* with a woman's body."

I had come to interview Dr. Northrup for an article on the connection between a woman's health and her wealth, but as we settled in her office, the conversation naturally turned to relationships and starting a family. "My husband would like to have children," I told her, "and for the first time in my life, I actually feel that I may be ready for a child. I am a late bloomer, I guess, as I am in my 40s now." She nodded and told me about one of her best friends, whose mother had her at age 42 back in the fifties and who married the man of her dreams at 40. Dr. Northrup removed this woman's intrauterine device in a beautiful ritual, and together they called in a baby soul. Within three months, her friend was pregnant at 41.

"I totally get it," I said. "My own mother was 42 when she had me, and my grandmother was also 42 when she had her second child in 1945."

Dr. Northrup laughed. "Therefore, that is what your biology learned from your mother. You will get pregnant immediately. You will have no problems, and you will deliver like you are 21. That is the way it works, as this is your programming."

Curiously, this is exactly what happened when I was 44 years old.

"When I was a resident at St. Margaret's hospital for women in Boston, I was doing obstetrics," she continued. "The only way to get the Catholic Irish women to stop having babies was to perform a hysterectomy. We needed to do major surgery to stop them. Because, think about it—everybody around them was having children, and some of the women I saw at the hospitals were 45, 46, 47 when they had their babies. Why?"

I leaned forward, shrugging my shoulders.

"Because nobody told them they could not have babies in their 40s or that their eggs were old and not viable anymore. Nobody put a ticking time bomb inside their brain, which then affects their biology. So, their bodies went ahead and created more Catholic babies. I saw it all the time."

"So, for you, becoming a mother is not a question of age?" I asked.

"Not at all, because chronologic age and biologic age can be twenty years apart. Bettina, your biologic age is probably 30 or 32. Now, let's line you up with a bunch of other 40-year-olds, and here is what you would find: some look 60; some look 30—there is a huge range. Even if follicle stimulating hormone (FSH) and luteinizing hormone (LH) were up in the menopausal range, you could change your diet, you could change your thoughts, and you could get pregnant like Julia Indichova did and chronicled in her book *Inconceivable*.

"The fertility industry is so lucrative, we've made every woman over the age of 35 feel old, high-risk, and sub-fertile, believing it's 'never gonna happen.' When, in fact, some of the studies done on fertility were done on French Huguenots in the 1600s. The data on women's chances to conceive over 35 is wrong."

I fell silent for a moment, trying to process what she just said.

Dr. Northrup continued. "Society puts too much pressure on women to have children before a certain age. What is happening now is that women who are in their mid-30s and older have so many stress hormones from just hearing that they are too old, that their epinephrine and cortisol levels are already high, which interferes with the hypothalamic-pituitary-adrenal axis. Many women have already talked themselves out of it before they even try to conceive. And because their uterus and their brains are so profoundly connected, women are making themselves infertile but don't even know it. The more left-hemisphere dominant you get, the more MBAs and PhDs you have, the higher up the food chain you are, the worse it gets."

Your Thoughts and Beliefs Have a Real Impact on Your Body

Looking back, I think it was fate that I brought this topic up long before I conceived my child, let alone this book. "Women are making themselves infertile but don't even know it" was the sentence that I never forgot from my conversation with Dr. Northrup, as it hit so close to home for me. The extraordinarily strong mind-body connection has been scientifically well established for quite some time now, yet this intrinsic bond between my thoughts and my self-talk and my physical well-being was never as vivid to me than when I experienced my own fertility challenges. I actually had previously done exactly what Dr. Northrup had said: inhibited my fertility without being aware of it.

When Joshua and I ditched the contraceptives for one whole year, I was riddled with ambivalence about having a child. My heart had already said yes, but my mind, my ever-so-smart and crazy, non-stop, chattering mind, came up with a slew of reasons as to why this was not a good idea.

Today, I know that I was ruled by fear. I had overanalyzed my situation and listened only to my intellect and nothing else. I was focusing on the limitations a child would bring into my life and how my life would change for the worse. This stressed me out in precisely the way Dr. Northrup mentioned, pumping stress hormones into my system that inhibited my female wonderland, everything from my fallopian tubes to my uterus, from working as it was designed to. (As a side note, the uterus in Traditional Oriental medicine is aptly called the palace your future child will reside in.) My mind had spoken, and my body had shelved my fertility accordingly.

Now, my incessant fears and negative self-talk were unique to me and my personal struggles, but there are plenty of other dreads and worries that many of us mature women have and often focus on:

- "I am too old; I've squandered my chances to have a child."
- "My eggs are not good anymore; I need to do IVF right away."
- "I was told by my doctor that I am infertile. I am infertile!"
- "Nobody understands what infertility does to a woman."
- "My body will fail; I know it."
- "Something will go wrong, just like it did for my sister and my best friend. I am sure of it."
- "I will miscarry again. My body is not strong enough anymore."
- "I will never have the child I so much long for."
- "How can I be a good mother when I have such bad memories and imprints from my own family?"
- "A satisfying career and a loving family at the same time—I don't think that's possible."
- "My mother almost died giving birth to my brother. What will delivery do to me?"

Decide for yourself if negative thoughts and beliefs, left unresolved, could have an impact on a woman's body.

When I conducted the interviews for my book, I realized that many of the women I spoke to had some thought patterns and deep-seated beliefs to overcome before pregnancy, whether they were conscious of them at first or not. Claudia Spahr (chapter 13) lost her very first pregnancy and doubted her body was strong enough to carry a child to term. Larissa (chapter 9) thought her upbringing by alcoholic parents rendered her unfit to become the kind of mother she wanted to be for her own child. Ellen (chapter 6) had locked a traumatic experience so deep inside her body that she never ovulated or menstruated until she uncovered the real reason for her polycystic ovary syndrome (PCOS). Leah (chapter 4) lost five pregnancies before she discovered cognitive hypnotherapy and uncovered her mental blocks. And Jenny (chapter 5) got herself so worked up by fear that she would never have a family and the child she so longed for, that she ended up being hospitalized for six weeks at an inpatient facility off the coast of England.

You will read about all these women and more. All of them went on to naturally conceive one, two, even three healthy children in their 40s because they had awareness, courage, and bravery. It meant taking time and slowing down—the total opposite of "quick, quick, your clock is ticking!" pressure we get from most doctors—to work out their mental "stuff" before welcoming new children into this world. It has been scientifically proven that the brain does not function isolated from the immune, endocrine, nervous, and other systems in your body. Today, mind/body research is confirming what ancient healing traditions have always known: the body and the mind are a unit, and there is no disease where there isn't a mental and emotional component as well as physical. So be very *mindful* of that.

All of us had our doubts and deep beliefs to overcome, and I definitely had my fair share of them as well. Curiously though, the fear that my body could not handle the challenge of conception and pregnancy in my 40s never came up. Not even once. I have never heard my biological clock tick—not even now, at almost 47. My career clock has ticked like crazy since I turned 42, yes, but my biological clock has not yet. Why? Because I consciously choose what I believe in and what is true for me—that I am strong, healthy, and teeming with fertility in my 40s—instead of falling in line with what most other people are believing or repeating because they heard others say so. And I encourage you wholeheartedly to also become very vigilant about your beliefs around your own fertility and to change them if they don't support you. I am not saying that you should just "snap out of it" and from now on believe that you are super-duper fertile. That would be silly of me to suggest, and it would not work for you. What I am saying, though, is this:

- Become aware of what you believe around your fertility. Really contemplate what you trust to be true, who influenced your beliefs, what stories shaped your beliefs, etc. Identify your deep beliefs and own them.
- Then ask yourself: Is what I believe really true and 100 percent set in stone and unchangeable? Or do I have evidence that a different belief— backed up by new information I previously might not have had—would serve me better and bring me closer to my desired outcome? Can I get behind shifting my belief?
- If so, *choose* the belief that will support you better on your path and choose it every single day. Do it not because anybody else told you to do it (including me), but because it is more supportive of the life you want to create *regardless* of what others tell you.
- Make it a daily practice to consciously choose your beliefs—especially if (or when) you catch yourself falling back into old thought patterns. This daily choice of beliefs is tremendously important once you are aware of how much we are influenced, not just by individuals but by society itself.

Now let's have a look around and see how our culture influences our beliefs and, subsequently, our biology. Our bodies are influenced and actually structured by our thoughts and beliefs. Every thought is accompanied by an emotion or feeling, and every emotion creates a specific biochemical reality in our bodies.

Thoughts that are reinforced over and over again become beliefs. Beliefs drive behaviors.

Have you noticed how our culture collectively conforms to certain beliefs and turns them into "truths" that most of us adhere to? There are the beliefs that are more general, like, "Women have to be a certain dress size to be beautiful"; "You'll never be successful if you don't finish college"; or, "I can't get ahead because of the economy." On a more personal level, it's, "Nature intended that women have children early"; "I just don't have the energy anymore that I used to have ten years ago"; or, "Getting older is not for the faint of heart."

We Are All Products of Our Culture

One woman, Pippa (chapter 11), had tried for seven years—from age 35 to 42—to conceive with her husband, David. It was not until she started working with Traditional Chinese medicine practitioner and fertility expert Andrew Loosely that she overcame one of the biggest mental imprints most of us have to overcome: the idea that we are physically too old to have a child in our 40s. "In Chinese medicine, which is a five-thousand-year-old science, a woman can have children until menopause," Pippa told me after she naturally conceived her son only seven months (!) after working with Andrew. There is no stigma around later motherhood in China. There is no tight timeline or pressure to be done by 35—or 45. Unfortunately, we women in the Western world are not so lucky, and we literally, not just figuratively, embody our cultural beliefs.

Through Dr. Northrup's book *Goddesses Never Age* (I highly recommend this resource), I was introduced to the fascinating work of Dr. Mario Martinez, founder of the Biocognitive Institute, which bridges the field of psychoneuroimmunology, cultural anthropology, and cultural neuroscience. Dr. Martinez is a clinical neuropsychologist who lectures worldwide on the impact of cultural beliefs on health and longevity. He is also the author of the book *The Mind Body Code*. Dr. Martinez wondered what would happen with our immune system when a word with cultural weight—which, arguably, the word "infertility" carries—enters our bio-informational field. He found that, in overt and subtle ways, our cultural beliefs impact our immune system. Several studies indicate that shame, for example, causes inflammation.

Here's a captivating example of his findings: In Peru and other South American countries, *bochorno* is the word used for the hot flashes of menopause. In Spanish, *bochorno* means "shame." In Japan, on the other hand, hot flashes are called *konenki*, which means "change or turn of life," and in Chinese medicine, menopause is considered a "second spring" (as Pippa surely also knows). I was fascinated to read that South American women who experience their hot flashes as shame have significantly more inflammatory problems and painful symptoms. They are more likely to need hormone replacement therapy and experience a diminished sense of beauty than their Japanese and Chinese counterparts, who welcome menopause as a natural transition to the second spring of their lives.

Dr. Martinez argues that, in general, our biology adjusts to our cultural beliefs and that, in particular, our immune system confirms how we choose to view the world. In other words: the hope of a second spring is a very powerful immune enhancer, but the helplessness women experience with a shameful hot flash is a very powerful immune detractor. Think about this.

I suggest you erase the word "infertility" completely from your vocabulary, regardless of whether you already experience challenges or just expect you will. It's not a good word as it smacks of failure and shame and, as you now know, can cause serious negative impact on your well-being. Stop using this word; stop searching for articles with this keyword; stop looking to your mother, sister, or best friend for reasons to believe your own body could be broken. Even if—or *especially* if—a person of authority, like a doctor, told you that you are infertile, do *not* think of yourself like that. Do not take on this label and use it for self-punishment and loathing self-talk.

We all have a tendency to be our own worst enemy and to speak to ourselves in a way we would never speak about a friend or someone we loved. Words are tremendously powerful and carry a charge that can uplift you or bring you down. Shaming words cause inflammation and possibly painful symptoms, which are the last things you want when you're trying to conceive a healthy baby. Make sure to read the Action Steps at the end of this pillar for suggestions on how to nourish your mind and uplift your body.

If Cultural Beliefs Can Impact Our Bodies, Can a Change in Belief Reverse the Impact?

What can happen if you take people out of their culture and put them into a controlled environment? Or, if you change their mindset about their perceived reality? In studies conducted over four decades, Harvard psychology professor Ellen Langer—a creative social scientist without any respect for conventional wisdom—showed that mental attitude can reverse the effects of aging and improve physical health. Some of her earlier work includes the famous Counterclockwise Study, which the *New York Times Magazine* devoted large parts to in "What if Age Is Nothing but a Mindset?"

"One day in the fall of 1981," Bruce Grierson writes in this article, "eight men in their 70s stepped out of a van in front of a converted monastery in New Hampshire. They shuffled forward, a few of them arthritically stooped, a couple with canes. Then they passed through the door and entered a time warp. Perry Como crooned on a vintage radio. Ed Sullivan welcomed guests on a black-and-white TV. Everything inside —including the books on the shelves and the magazines lying around —were designed to conjure 1959."

The men were asked to bring their suitcases to their rooms themselves, even if it meant carrying one shirt at a time. For one week, the experimental group was surrounded by paraphernalia from twenty years earlier, listening to radio shows and discussing news from that period. They were not allowed to talk about anything past 1959, and they were told to refer to themselves, their careers, and their families as they would have twenty-two years earlier. Before arriving, the men were assessed on such measures as dexterity, grip strength, flexibility, hearing and vision, memory and cognition. By simply behaving like men decades younger for less than a week, the change in the group was remarkable: the men showed improvements in "physical strength, manual dexterity, gait, posture, perception, memory, cognition, taste sensitivity, hearing, and vision." A couple of men, who had seemed frail only a few days ago, even engaged in an impromptu touch football game on the front lawn.

In another study, the Hotel Maid Study, which I find to be especially mindboggling, Dr. Langer spoke to chambermaids and asked them if they got enough exercise. Surprisingly, the majority said no, even though they were physically active all day long, from changing sheets to scrubbing bath tubs and hauling vacuum cleaners around. Langer took several measures of the women's basic fitness levels, which indicated that they, indeed, had the poor health of basically sedentary people. Then she divided eighty-four chambermaids into two groups and gave one group a new perspective on their work.

The maids were told that cleaning fifteen rooms every day constitutes more than enough activity to meet the surgeon general's recommendation of a half-hour of daily physical activity. The researcher even provided calorie counts for specific tasks and posted this new perspective and truth in the maids' quarters in the hotels for them to see and be reminded. The other group was given no such information.

Only one month later, the study-group maids had lost two pounds on average, saw their systolic blood pressure drop by ten points, and were "significantly healthier" overall. Think about it: the women did not change their behavior, just their mindset! Now that they believed they exercised daily, their bodies followed suit. "Wherever you put the mind, you're necessarily putting the body," Dr. Langer explained in a recent *CBS This Morning* interview.

When you believe that something will affect you in a particular way, it often does. That's why every rigorous clinical trial includes placebo controls, which we will dive into deeper in the BODY section. Your own expectations, and the expectations of others, are powerful. Unfortunately, expectations of the declining cognitive and physical abilities that come with age are pervasive (we'll also touch more on the topic of chronological age versus biological age in the BODY pillar).

Ageism Is Intense: Are You Guilty of It Yourself?

Now, let me ask you a crucial question: what do you believe about your age? Your beliefs are actually stronger than your genes, and yes, that is scientifically proven.

So, what do you truly believe? Do you believe that your reproductive organs know that you turned 35 or 40, so they now need to deteriorate? Do you believe your body will know to stop functioning effectively at a certain age? Do you believe you are simply getting older or that you are aging and declining? In America, women face intense ageism—are you guilty of this yourself? How do you talk about your age? Are you blaming health problems on your age? Are you saying things like, "Now that I am older, I just don't have the energy anymore to do XYZ"? Are you using your age to avoid attention? Or to draw attention? Are you using your age as an excuse to not show up fully? Pay attention to the words you use about growing older and the meaning you give those words. Until you bring these beliefs to the forefront of your consciousness, they can have a significant adverse effect on your health.

My advice is to stop thinking about your age and, ideally, stop talking about your age as well. It's funny how often I observe people adapting their attitude toward me once they know I am older than they expected me to be. On a good day (also known as the day after plenty of sleep), with a little makeup and a good blow dry, I can still pass as in my mid-30s. And having a toddler at that age is normal and well accepted by society. But wait until people find out that I am actually a decade older—they usually stare at me for a second and then at my boy before saying things like, "You got really lucky to have a healthy son at your age," or, "I would never have the energy to deal with a little child at that age; I am so happy I had mine early," or, "You look great *for your age*," or, and I am not kidding, "Good thing there are fertility treatments" (actually said to me by a man in his 50s), or, *the* classic, "Are you a mom or grandmom?"

Why? Because there is this opaque yet widespread picture in most peoples' heads of what being 46 looks like, what it means in terms of aging and deterioration, and what it means when it comes to fertility and vitality. On one of my first outings with my newborn, Hunter, I ran into a lovely lady from the

South at a farmers market in Virginia (I was 44). She was very happy to consider me as my boy's mother until my age came up in conversation, and I literally turned into a grandmother before her eyes. It had nothing to do with me or my looks but everything to do with her and her conditioning of what a number means. We all have these unwritten imprints.

I, myself, sometimes find myself in disbelief that I am nearing 50 whenever I am unconsciously letting my imprint run the show. And even though I am much more mindful now about my own self-talk and my imprints, I still find myself from time to time judging other peoples' age based on a number. (Curiously, they are usually much older than me, even if they are younger.) As a side note, I am with Dr. Northrup when she suggests in *Goddesses Never Age* to stop celebrating milestone birthdays after, say, 30 or 33. It makes sense when you know how a number shapes the perspective of others, as well as your own perspective! If I had not been writing a book for which my age actually matters, I, indeed, would have become ageless by now.

What we choose to believe affects how we deal with our world, and we construct our world based on what we perceive with our culturally trained brain. If you think you are old, you will behave differently than if you think you are not, as Dr. Langer's experiments proved. If you believe that the world is a malevolent, hostile place, you will find more proof for that assumption than a person who thinks the world is benevolent. A fertility specialist will most likely passionately argue that a woman's reproductive system is in decline after 40 because he sees it on a daily basis in his office and he reads all about infertility in his industry-specific ART media.

Remember the report "Infertility in America 2015" by the Reproductive Medicine Associates of New Jersey that I mentioned in the introduction? From a PR standpoint (I was once the head of communication for a New York City hedge fund and know good public relations when I see it), it was brilliantly written, and it suggested that the Millennial generation will automatically seek out fertility treatments as ART will be the new normal. So, a fertility specialist will argue that fertility drops after 35, free falls after 40, and that egg quality diminishes because he sees it and reads it all the time, and therefore, it's the truth.

It's his reality also because the healthy women who are fully fertile later into their 40s would not go and seek his services. His world is full of infertility.

My reality is that women in their 40s are blossoming mothers in their prime. That's what I saw growing up, what I've experienced myself as a vibrant mother, and what I've found in my conversations with more than sixty women over 40 with whom I easily crossed paths for this book. I've witnessed it in my circle of friends, the women I've met in Hunter's preschool, in my extended professional circles, and in my own family. I've also seen it in the success stories of the dozen natural fertility experts I've interviewed, many of whom can claim a much higher success rate than most fertility clinics. There is *a lot* more fertility in our 40s than we hear about and are led to believe.

Both perspectives, that of fertility experts and of fertile women over 40, are "real," and we have "reality" to back it all up. And I am passionately arguing that both perspectives are just as valid and it's time to shift the doom and gloom narrative to one that is more balanced, equally truthful, and real. I believe it's about time to have a concerted discussion about later motherhood, and I think it's about time for us women to take back responsibility for our health and our fertility.

Yet, the most important question concerning your fertility is this: **what do *you* choose to believe and welcome into your life?**

CHAPTER 2

Let's Honor Our Female Ancestors

Women in Their 40s Have Birthed Children under All Circumstances

Before I started researching this book, I hadn't thought much about the countless generations of women who had birthed children for thousands and thousands of years long before it was my turn. I had not much considered our female ancestors who had ensured the continuum of human life on earth. Why would I? Giving birth to babies happens every single second of every single day all around the world. According to UNICEF, there are 353,000 children born each day, which is 4.3 births every second. Having babies is normal; nothing special really, is it?

I was naïve and did not realize the magnitude of motherhood until I became a mother myself. I had not really grasped that in the moment a baby makes its first cry (or, sadly, not), a mother is born. A mother is born in all her love, with all her flaws and her lifelong dedication to her child. Today, I am aware that every single woman who ever conceived a child in the history of mankind would also have had a story to tell. She had emotions to share and often heartache to unburden. Maybe she was isolated from other women or, if lucky, warmly embedded in the community of sisterhood. She may have lived in a mountain village or next to the ocean. Perhaps she was married to a man who worshiped her or to one who violated her. If she was famous, the history books might tell a little of her, but most likely, her story was never captured, and she's been forgotten as if she never existed.

Yet, we cannot talk about conceiving children and bearing babies without recognizing and paying respect to the women in our lineage whose joy, pain, and dedication made it possible for us to be born and thrive. None of us would be here were it not for our mothers, grandmothers, and all the other women throughout our lineage who birthed the next generation. There is a good chance—actually, I think it's a certainty—that you, yourself, had multiple female ancestors who conceived children in their 40s and bore them under circumstances much different from those today. Please go and ask your mother, aunts, or any female elder you can find in your family to shed some light on your female lineage, to tell of all the women who overcame and endured and loved and fought and held their children close. Finally hearing their stories may give you valuable clues to who you are and what you are capable of.

My Family's Fertility Story

I am the third generation of women who had children in their 40s, but I expect there were many more before. Most of my female ancestors grew up in Europe in an area that was once part of the Roman Empire, later known as the Austrian-Hungarian empire until World War I, and which is now Austria, a country of 8.5 million people. My maternal grandparents were modest people. My grandfather worked for the railroad company, and my grandmother, whom we called Oma, was a homemaker. My Oma, Hermine, had one daughter, my mother, Susanne, at age 26, and her second child, my aunt Hermi, when she was 42 years old. It was an unplanned pregnancy, as has surely happened in every single lineage throughout time.

Unfortunately, my grandfather had only wanted to have one child and blamed my grandmother for becoming pregnant with Hermi. Yes, he blamed her for having fallen pregnant with his child. He was so furious with his wife that this otherwise decent and kind man supposedly never touched her again. I can hardly imagine what mixed feelings my grandmother must have felt about the baby that was growing in her belly.

When the time came to give birth, Oma knew that she needed to walk to the hospital, but she did not know if she'd survive the journey. While her husband was, to put it mildly, unsupportive, the timing of her second birth was even worse: it was early 1945, a few months before the end of WWII. By that time, the Allied forces flew air raids over Vienna, dropping bombs that left death and rubble in their wake. When labor started, my grandmother walked all by herself to the nearest hospital. Twice she had to seek shelter when the terrifying alarm sounded, signaling the approach of hundreds of airplanes whose mission was to shower the city with bombs. She waited underground, in labor, to see if the building above her would be hit.

Twice her life was spared, and she somehow made her way out onto the streets again, where people rushed home to their loved ones or dug for them underneath the debris. In the chaos, I doubt anybody noticed the laboring woman, let alone helped her. Eventually my grandmother made it to the hospital. When the next attack came, the nurse left her alone and ran to save her own life. My grandmother was in the last stage of labor, unable to seek shelter. Finally, a young male doctor came and took mercy on her. "I will help you," he said, and he delivered my aunt, in spite of the bombing, and with nothing but his gloved hands and scissors.

There was no fetal heart monitor, no epidural, no medical team standing by if the baby should require intensive care or if the mother should hemorrhage. There was just the force of a baby wanting to be born and her mother's body that obliged. Having birthed my son at age 44, without any medication or medical intervention, but in a safe room in a safe city with dimmed lights and soothing music and my husband and a team of loving caregivers by my side, I cannot fathom how my Oma and my aunt did it practically alone amidst a raging war, all the while fearing that they could be buried under a collapsing building.

The human spirit is incredibly strong, and if a life is supposed to survive, it will. If you have any doubts that birthing a healthy child in your 40s is possible, remember Oma's story. You, yourself, have similar stories in your own lineage; I guarantee it.

Even after all she endured, my grandmother described being a mature mother as if it was the best thing that could have happened to her. "The 40s are the best decade in a woman's life," she'd say. "You know who you are and where the direction of your life leads you, and you are still young enough to fully enjoy your child and see it grow up." My grandparents' relationship may never have been the same, but both parents individually found profound joy and love in their relationship to their youngest daughter. Aunt Hermi became my grandfather's beloved darling, the apple of his eye, and Hermi was my Oma's biggest support and emotional pillar in her later and final years, after my grandfather had died and her health started to wane. If I could ask my grandmother if she would do it all again, she most likely would give me a resounding yes.

An Interview with My Mother

My mother, too, speaks highly of her experience as an older mom, but you better not use that term in front of her. "I always saw myself as younger than my age, and even today, I often forget how old I really am," she told me when I interviewed her for this book. We sat in my mom's living room in my childhood home outside of Vienna. Mami, as I call her, is now 89 years old and still smart as a whip. She's been living by herself since the night my father passed away in August of 2003, and she still manages all of her daily life, either by herself or with some help from my older brother. My parents were married for fifty-two years and had their own triumphs and tragedies on their way to parenthood. They experienced eight (!) miscarriages. Every time, the pregnancy was far enough along for them to be able to tell that all the babies were boys. I was child number ten, the second one to survive, and the only girl.

I have to look at my mother's youth to understand how she could endure eight miscarriages without falling into despair, being overcome by grief, or simply going crazy. Mami was 10 years old when Adolf Hitler marched into Vienna and annexed Austria to Germany and 17 when WWII ended. For her, a smart, gorgeous, and well-aware teenager with blonde hair and steel-blue eyes, these years were formative. My mother knows what hunger and winter cold feels like when there isn't any wood to burn in the stove—"The relentless cold is much worse than hunger"—and she knows the fear of potentially dying in a bombing raid and the terror of hiding in the hay up in the attic of their farmhouse while Russian soldiers raped her mother one story below.

These imprints don't lose their grip on a person, especially not for a generation of people who frowned upon seeking psychological help. My parents never saw a therapist for what they went through. "The war" was often a topic of conversation during my childhood. And it had, as I now understood, steeled both my parents for their "fertility challenges."

In her own words, Susanne, my mother: I studied at the University of Vienna under really difficult circumstances. Your father and I were poor. I was only one of two women at the whole University. My parents were very supportive, especially my father, but they had very limited funds to give me. It was the time after WWII, when students needed to pay money in order to take one of the big exams. So instead of having money for food that week, we starved so I could take the test. Once I had my degree and was a biochemist, I wanted to work and make a professional impact. At first, having babies did not fit my life's plan.

None of my children were planned; they just came. We were newlyweds and 23 years old when I got pregnant for the first time. I had terrible morning sickness, as I subsequently had with all my pregnancies, but everything was fine until blood started to gush out of me when I was about six or seven months along. Your father took me to the hospital, but our OB/GYN was not there yet. A nurse gave me an injection to get my labor going, but my doctor never made it in time.

I birthed our first son with extremely painful contractions but without anybody's help, as the nurses were not allowed to deliver—they had to wait for the doctor. Basically, only your father was there. I lost so much blood, it went through the mattress and pooled underneath my bed. When I looked at the boy I had birthed, it was uncanny to see how much this child looked like your father. It was unbelievable—he even had your dad's big hands and long fingers. I believe he was already dead when he was born, but I am not 100 percent sure.

Bettina: You don't even know if he was alive?

No, there was nobody there to check on him. It was very sad. Your dad held it together for me while I was in the hospital. But my sister, Hermi, told me many years later that he broke down at home in front of her and cried and cried, repeating, "We lost the child." I mourned, too, deeply. But a few days later, I needed to go back to work, and thankfully, my job offered a much-needed distraction from what just happened. My work offered solace, and in a twist of fate, it was also most likely the culprit for all of the losses.

Your father and I were young, healthy, and both very fertile. I got pregnant easily. Besides the morning sickness, things would be fine until the bleeding started. My gynecologist would usually order me to stay home on bed rest for two or three weeks, and all would be fine. Then I'd go back to work on a Monday, and by the next weekend, I would lose the pregnancy, and nobody could tell me why! My doctors always said that I had a great female anatomy, a great uterus, perfect hips—physically, everything was right. They did some hormonal tests and blood tests, but nothing led to a real explanation as to why I miscarried so often.

Your brother, Martin, was my seventh pregnancy. I was 32 by that time, and I really wanted to have a child. I stayed on bed rest for most of the pregnancy, and he was the first boy that I carried to term. We both almost died during delivery, but that's another story. The doctors were elated and said that now I had carried one pregnancy to term, I could have ten more children if I wanted. They were wrong. The next two pregnancies also ended in miscarriage.

It was not until many years later, when I read an American scientific study published in one of the medical journals that had studied women who were chemists and were pregnant, that I finally understood. By then, scientists had discovered that certain chemical reactions produced fumes that interfered with a woman's hormones. I am simplifying now, but basically, these fumes give the body the signal to get rid of the foreign object. The mother's body got the signal "repel!" and her body miscarried accordingly.

My office was right next to the laboratory. Even though I was not inside the laboratory producing these poisonous fumes myself, I was exposed to them in such quantity that I lost all the pregnancies. In hindsight, it makes total sense. Now I know why I miscarried within days of going back to work, but at that time, we simply did not know what was going on.

How did you not fall into despair or become overwhelmed by grief after losing eight children?

Bettina, if you survived the war, you were just lucky to be alive. What we went through is impossible for your generation to comprehend. At first it was not so bad, as we had the farm outside of Vienna and a little food and heating material, but it got bad in the later years. You'd wake up in the morning, thinking that today you may die. It was most horrible when the bombs dropped on Vienna and you were close to a building that collapsed. We all tried to rescue survivors, and I remember digging for them. I remember listening for knocking sounds, as that was the way the survivors could communicate with those of us above ground. They would tap on a pipe to make themselves heard. And it was most horrible if we finally got to them, but it was too late, and everybody was dead. The old people, the young, children, the little babies—all either suffocated or were struck to death, and maybe only one was still able to tap on a pipe.

We had a small bag with our documents, and every time I ran into the shelters with my mother and baby sister, I prayed, "Dear God, if it needs to be today, then please take us quickly. Don't let us suffer." One day my mother was not with us, and I was alone with Hermi when the sirens started to warn us of the coming air raid. Hermi was so small she just lay on the kitchen table. I was 16 and did not know what to do. I threw myself over her and cried that she should not be afraid, that we'd die together.

When you experience life like that, you become hard. You become really tough. *(Mami and I, we were both crying by now.)* Your mindset becomes very focused: I am still alive, so I will still be okay, even after the miscarriages. Your father and I knew we would still be okay, regardless of whether we became parents or not. We would be okay—and were happy, regardless of our losses.

Eventually you brought one boy to term. And then, ten years later, at age 41, you skipped a period again.

Yes, I was convinced I was in menopause. After losing yet another boy, I was done. I told your father that I was done. I really did not want to do it anymore. So, I went to the doctor to have him confirm that I was in menopause. And he told me that I was pregnant again. I must admit, it was a bit of a shock. I struggled with the knowledge. I quit smoking and drinking, but I also told your father that I would not stay on bed rest anymore. Luckily, I had changed jobs by then and was no longer exposed to the toxic fumes.

The pregnancy actually was good and much different from the experience with your brother, Martin, a decade earlier. The way the doctors approached pregnancy had changed. While they had suggested bed rest with Martin, I was now encouraged to go for walks and even do light exercise. They were not worried about my age, or at least I don't remember them to be. At some point, I contracted a tapeworm after eating meat that was not cooked well enough. I had to take medication to expel that thing, which was also dangerous for you, the unborn fetus. The medication could have brought on a miscarriage, but you hung on and were not deterred *(laughing)*.

But when I contracted the Spanish flu and had a major coughing fit in my seventh month of pregnancy, my water broke five weeks before your due date. It happened in the middle of a snowstorm in January, and your father and I drove to two different hospitals before finally being admitted. Within two hours of the arrival of my doctor, you were born. He administered a combination of labor-inducing medication as well as a pain reliever, and the birth was so much easier than your brother's birth ten years earlier. You were small, only 5.5 pounds, but healthy. Unfortunately, I still had a high fever, and they were understaffed at this hospital because of the Spanish flu. So, you were taken from me and brought to a children's hospital right away because you needed to be in the incubator for a couple of days. I was not allowed to hold you, and I did not see you again for two whole weeks.

I was not with you or any other family member for the first two weeks of my life?

No, unfortunately not. I know this would not happen today.

How was later motherhood for you?

Totally normal. Since my mother had Hermi at age 42, it seemed absolutely natural to me to be the same age when I delivered you. I always looked a bit younger, and so I think people usually did not know how old I was. Naturally, we made friends with the parents of your friends, and they were often ten or fifteen years younger. I am friends with some of them still today, and even now they attest that they never saw an age difference between themselves and your father and me.

And, the truth is, having a child in your 40s is a fountain of youth—if you choose to keep up with the demands of your child. Sure, we could have put you in front of the TV a lot so we could relax and be sedentary ourselves, but that's not what we wanted for you. We wanted you to be healthy and play. If a man and a woman choose to have a child later in life, I believe they need to choose to be active themselves and do whatever it takes to stay healthy and agile for the next eighteen years and beyond. That's our responsibility as older parents to our children.

We always did whatever our much younger friends did with their kids, like going hiking or camping, or swimming in lakes in the summer. We did not say, "Sorry, we are too old for that," and so age was never a topic of concern. In fact, when friends that were our age, in their 50s, started to complain about ailments, we still went cross-country skiing with you, despite the fact that neither one of us were particularly athletic. Well, your father more than I. Instead of talking about illnesses with our peers, we engaged in whatever was going on with our younger friends, which usually did not have to do with sickness.

However, this topic brings me to another point: one of my close friends, who is almost twenty years younger, lost her husband to cancer when their two children were under the age of 10. So, having children younger or older does not necessarily determine the amount of time you will have with them. I've also read that people who have children later in life stay physically healthier longer.

Yes, there are also now studies that attest that children of older parents are taller, stronger, and more educated than children of younger parents. And that, if a woman is able to conceive naturally after 35, she is four times more likely to live past 90.

Being 89 years old right now, I can attest to that. I am immensely grateful that I was able to see the evolution of Hunter and see how this tiny human being formed inside your body. Being able to see the ultrasound and watch how a human grows from a tiny spot on the screen into a full-fledged being, seeing how life evolves inside the mother's body—it's a miracle! I am so grateful for having had the chance to experience it, as this is so different from my own experience.

Hermi and I, we were both pregnant at the same time with our daughters, and we seriously thought that the baby wasn't alive until it was born. We did not have this connection to the baby inside our bodies. Strange, but that's how it was. It's also beautiful to see how different fatherhood has become. I don't remember that your father ever touched my pregnant belly or changed your diaper or soothed you to sleep. It's heartwarming for me to see how Joshua was involved in every aspect of his son's life.

Do you regret being an older grandparent? At 89, you don't have the physical strength and stamina anymore to keep a super-active 3-year-old in check. Do you see this as a negative? Do you wish we would have had Hunter sooner?

24

I don't wish that you and Joshua would have had Hunter earlier, because the timing was right for the two of you. The timing must be right for the parents, not the grandparents. If you two would have had Hunter any earlier, would you have awaited him with so much love? I don't know. But I remember that Joshua and you were very deliberate and debated for a long time if you should even have children. You two were very conscious about having a child, and then you said yes before even trying—and did it at an age when it is not so common anymore. Your child was wanted from the first second on, and that is something special, and it is because the timing was right for you. And so, it is right for Hunter, me, and everybody else.

Would you recommend having a child past 40?

Yes! Because by then you know yourself, and you know where your life is headed. You are more conscious of what it means to have a child and of what it means to guide another human being in the first two decades of his or her life. You understand, at least somewhat, that you need to leave things behind that you can no longer do as a parent because of the responsibility you choose to take on. These are all really good things for the parents to know before they have a baby, and it is also good for the child.

I also think that when you are as old as I am, you will ask yourself, "What meaning did my life have?" That question will come, whether you embrace it or not. Will what you have worked for and what you have built be given to the next generation? Or will it end up in a public trust and you'll be completely forgotten? I see it in the old ladies at church who have nobody now that their spouses have passed away. Their lives have become meaningless, and some of them even say so.

Of course, I know that there can be insurmountable rifts within families, but in general, if you have children, you have a loving bond with them. You have somebody to look after you, to say, "I like you," or to give you a hug when you are old and widowed. Who is left in old age but your children? Will you look back at your life and think about how you raised your child or the awesome vacation you took? You may not have thought about that, Bettina, but I do. And

I cannot tell you how immensely grateful I am for having had my children who now look after me. So, yes, I would encourage women to say yes to life!

CHAPTER 3

Aimee

When I researched this book, my home office looked like the backroom of a Barnes and Noble: stacks and stacks of books on pregnancy, fertility, and longevity were scattered around, making it difficult for my rambunctious toddler to just sweep through the room in chase of our dog (no worries, she's a sixty-pound Pit Bull mix—she can hold her own). Any book you can find on Amazon relating to pregnancy, I most likely have it somewhere in my piles.

However, one of the books immediately stood out for me, and I can find it a heartbeat: Aimee Raupp's *Yes, You Can Get Pregnant*. Aimee is a recognized expert in Traditional Oriental medicine, acupuncture, and Chinese herbalism. She runs highly successful private clinics in New York City, the Hamptons, and Nyack, New York, all adorned with pictures of the hundreds, possibly thousands, of babies that she helped bring into this world through her practice, book, and online presence.

Aimee is a raven-haired woman whose beauty is unassuming, like a sister who does not need to show off to stand in her power and feel beautiful herself. Just listening to a video intro on her website made me feel like I really wanted to meet this woman and that we would totally hit it off. In her book, Aimee takes readers on her fertility-rejuvenation protocol, as she calls it, and she does it with a voice of authority and love for the women who come to her. She speaks of the uterus as the "palace where the child resides" and discusses how this palace is connected to the heart and the kidney. Aimee prescribes diet, herbs, and supplements, as well as courage, passion, and joy to enhance fertility.

Naturally, I reached out to Aimee to interview her as one of my experts for this book. And guess what? I got a two-for-one deal—both an expert and a mother—as Aimee had become a mother herself for the first time two days after her 41st birthday. At age 42, she was getting ready for a second baby. So, while her firstborn son slept happily in the adjacent room, Aimee and I hit the ground running during our Skype chat.

Bettina: First off, congratulations on your baby boy! You look very happy and content. Why did you wait so long to start your family?

I didn't find the right guy any sooner; that's it, plain and simple. I've wanted to become a mother for at least ten years now. And I did have good men in my life, but they were not husband material, at least not for me. It just was not quite right, you know? But I believed in divine timing and that, eventually, I would meet the man who would become my husband and the father of my child. So, I did not compromise, and I didn't settle, which I am very grateful for. I was very clear on what I wanted—not in a rigid way but in a way that honored myself. Looking back, I strongly feel that I met my husband exactly at the correct time.

Talk to me about that. How did you keep your faith throughout your 30s, all the while helping others to successfully get pregnant?

I used the time to work on myself and grow into the person, the mother, I am today. I had a life coach who helped me mature and helped me through the difficult times when my beloved father fell ill and eventually died. Back then, I was still in an immature stage, insecure, and maybe blaming others for where I was in my life, versus realizing that I was in control of how I felt and that I, alone, was responsible for my actions.

I also turned to teachers like Deepak Chopra, Gabrielle Bernstein, and other Hay House authors, and I listened to the teachings of people like Abraham Hicks. I had vision boards, and I kept journals. I would thank the universe in advance for delivering all the things I wanted to manifest. I did all sorts of things, which I continue to do by the way, because manifestations are real, and they are happening!

So, I tuned in to my internal dialogues and then shifted my belief system from being a victim to being empowered and in charge of how and what I felt, which was a big deal for me. I started to deeply love myself, and I came to trust the process. So, when I talk about self-love and trust to my clients, I truly can relate to their struggles and can help them find the love and trust in the process that they need.

Was it not difficult to see other women happily pregnant because of you, but you were not?

Not at all. In fact, I maintained my faith precisely because I saw women older than me getting pregnant all the time, and so I never really gave up. My mindset helped me here tremendously, as I think our reality is our perception. So, I chose to see the fertility all around me, and there is a lot more fertility than there is infertility! And there are a lot of women getting pregnant in their 40s. Was I without any doubt? No, of course not. I'd say that I was probably 85 percent sure all would work out fine. Sometimes fear crept up around maybe never finding the right guy. That was difficult for me, because I did not want to do it alone. I wanted a family and to make a baby out of love and bonding. So sometimes fear came, but I released it rather than holding on.

When did you meet your husband, and how quickly did you guys start the family planning?

We met a couple of months before my 40th birthday. We fell quickly and hard for each other, and after a few months together, it was clear to both of us that we were heading toward marriage. I turned 40 in September, and Ken suggested we get formally engaged around the holidays. I am very informal, so I said, "Sure, go ahead and plan it." I was more focused on getting pregnant by then.

"How long do you think it will take?" Ken asked. "Maybe six months," I answered. "Should I get my sperm checked?" I appreciated his openness because I know that, when couples have troubles conceiving, 50 percent of the time it's the man who is challenged. But by then I had Ken on my vitamin and mineral regimen and on a really healthy lifestyle for a few months already, and so there was really no reason for him to do that. I myself treated my body as a palace every day anyway, and my focus on health and nutrition came naturally. We got pregnant the second month we tried. Ken freaked out because he hadn't gotten the engagement ring yet, but I just laughed. I had always felt that I would get pregnant first and married second. Really, I've always felt that.

Your age was never a concern of yours?

No, never, because this is what I do for a living. I tell my patients all the time that they can improve their fertility. Age is just a chronological number, and your chronological age is very different from your biological age. I very much practice what I preach, and I follow my fertility rejuvenation protocol myself. Sure, the summer Ken and I met we were having a lot of fun, but I did not waiver in my nutrition, my supplements, my mindset, or the belief in my body, because I had seen it work for so many women I had helped.

Funnily enough, I had some people in my own practice who doubted my ability to get pregnant and were worried about my age. But I never did. I was very relieved, though, with how quickly it happened because I was like, "Oh, I really know what I am talking about." *(Laughing.)* It was so validating. One of my dear friends, who is very spiritual, once said to me, "This was God's will because he wanted you to have a baby at 40 because that's what you tell everyone that they can do. You had to do it at this age. You couldn't have done it before."

What do you say to a woman who confronts you with the statistics on age and fertility? Do you encourage her to just neglect the stats?

Allow me to quote from my own book about the statistics we so often read. In June of 2013, *The Atlantic* rebutted that age is our biggest deterrent to fertility. The story revealed that the widely cited statistic that one in three women, age 35 to 39, will not be pregnant after a year of trying is based on an article published in 2004 in the journal *Human Reproduction*. Rarely mentioned is the source of the data: French birth records from 1670 to 1830! No kidding. The chance of remaining childless—30 percent—was also calculated based on historical populations. In other words, millions of women are being told when to get pregnant based on statistics from a time before electricity, antibiotics, or fertility treatments. Most people assume these numbers are based on large, well-conducted studies of modern women, but they are not!

Just look around. Every woman reading this book may know other women in their late 30s and 40s who conceived healthy babies. I mean, your whole book is filled with such examples! Age is not the major issue here. The issue is much more complex. The process of getting pregnant is so multidimensional that, for one woman, it might just be a matter of having more timely sex; for another, it may be that she needs to change her diet; for another, it could be her chronic exposure to hormone-disrupting toxins in her shampoo or makeup; for another, it may be her husband's sperm; and another may have an autoimmune disease or all of the above.

And for yet another woman, it may be that she needs to work through her anger toward her mother. I am very serious here! In Traditional Oriental medicine, a five-thousand-year-old practice, the mental-emotional state of a woman is of utmost importance to her health and ability to conceive. And, by the way, we also see a lot of young couples having troubles conceiving nowadays for the same reasons mentioned above. Until you reach your mid-40s and late 40s, age is not the major issue getting pregnant. It's all the other things that factor into this delicate process.

Having lived in Manhattan myself for fourteen years, I am guessing you see a lot of successful, driven women in your New York City practice. What do you tell them when you first meet with them?

I ask them all the same question: do you really believe that you are going to have a baby? If they don't truly believe it, my work cannot be as effective. I tell them to not lose faith in their body and to realize that they have the power to change their health and affect their fertility. They have to trust where they are in the process and surrender. This is especially challenging for women working in male-dominated environments and women who are used to working hard and then getting what they set out to achieve. A tight mindset and often very tight timeline does not work in a woman's favor to conceive either. Women who are very controlling tend to be so because they lack trust and faith.

As a mental strength trainer, I could not agree more! People often don't realize how powerful their mind is and how their mind and focus influence their physiology.

I also tell all the women I work with that their fertility is an extension of their health, and so, when we improve their health, we improve their fertility. This is equally important to women who are using IVF as it is for women who want to conceive naturally. I want women going into IVF treatments to be as healthy as possible in order to boost their chances for the treatments to work and to ensure a healthy baby and a healthy pregnancy.

While I am working with women on the physical aspects, I also often need to boost their mental health as well. If a woman is anxious to start a family, she may have conversations in her head that are self-deprecating, where she is hard on herself and not loving. Of course, nobody walks around 100 percent totally in love with herself, but if a woman can think about herself and her body more than half the time in a loving and supportive way, it's enough to shift the energy. In my twelve years of treating more than four-hundred women one-on-one, only four did not get pregnant. Two adopted, one did not follow my program, and the fourth one is taking some time off right now. Traditional Oriental medicine is very powerful. And with all of my clients, I start with one mantra: I am where I am supposed to be, and I accept that.

What's the advantage or disadvantage of becoming a mom in your 40s?

I really can't answer that question fully because I've only been a 40+ mom, but I can tell you that I am very grateful for having done this in my 40s. On the one hand, I am hopeful that other women will see me as an inspiration and that this can be their paths as well. On the other hand, I am grateful because we women in our 40s are so much more evolved and in touch and in love with ourselves than we were when we were younger. We are, in general, in a place where we can treat our bodies and our lives with the respect they deserve. From that place, I can mother so much better!

This is what I preach to my clients in the clinic all the time: the more we can love ourselves, the better we are going to be as parents and as mothers. Then we won't put our problems onto our kids, which, unfortunately, plenty of parents do when they project their stuff onto the family unit. As older moms, we know that we are responsible for ourselves and that we need to take responsibility for our actions, our feelings, our emotions, our beliefs, our days. We need to be willing to see things differently and be willing to shift and change and honor our bodies and stop blaming others and stop blaming certain things. It's about taking back responsibility and power—and rocking it as a self-assured, mature mother!

CHAPTER 4

Leah

Leah Elliott's story made the rounds through the British newspapers two years ago with headlines like, "Woman Finally Gives Birth to Miracle Boy!" and I immediately understood why she drew so much attention. How *does* a woman not lose her hope for a healthy, natural pregnancy when, after losing one baby in the first trimester, she then goes on to lose another, after another, after another, after another? How *did* Leah, a slender beauty with long black hair and dark eyes, go through four and a half years of fertility struggles and come out of this dark period with her relationship intact and a healthy baby boy in her arms?

"I am not a person who gives up easily—I am quite the fighter," Leah told me when I reached her at her home in Stamford, an English town one-hundred miles north of London. "I threw myself into literature and studied infertility and general health, diet, and lifestyle. This research made me better understand how the body works and that I still had a good chance of conceiving and carrying a baby to full term again."

When Leah first met her partner, James, at a wedding, she was 33 years old. She did not worry about her fertility at first, as she already had a child—a daughter, conceived as quite a surprise at age 21—and figured that it may happen as easily again. However, that was not the case, and doubts about her age and her body's ability set in. The couple went through quite a roller coaster ride when she lost five pregnancies in almost as many years. Leah, devastated by the losses and also plagued by guilt surrounding her husband, James, who was six years younger, even contemplated letting go of the love of her life so he could, "go find somebody younger who could give him the child he wanted."

But James did not waver in his love, and the couple stayed on course. Over time, Leah changed her diet, changed her lifestyle, and even healed herself from Graves' disease, an autoimmune disorder. Then came the fateful weekend she paged through a magazine called *Fertility Road* and first read of Russell Davis, a cognitive hypnotherapist who specializes in fertility.

Russell, himself, had been in similar shoes before: he and his wife had overcome a decade of fertility struggles before finally conceiving their son naturally after being told they had a one-in-a-billion (!) chance of doing so. Leah and Russell started working together, and within four months, she was pregnant again. "This time it felt very different from the start." Leah credits the cognitive hypnotherapy for her easy pregnancy and her "miracle" baby, J.J., whom she was cradling in her arms at the hospital on her 40th birthday.

Bettina: When I first heard about you, Leah, I was not only impressed by your tenacity, but impressed that you and James were able to go through so much and come out of such hard times with your relationship intact, if not stronger. How did you do that?

Yes, these were very hard times. We started to try for a child about one-and-a-half years into our relationship, so we were fairly new into it. We were trying to navigate the waters of our committed relationship and at the same time deal with the joy of getting pregnant, with that joy soon turning into sadness and almost despair. The five miscarriages happened over a period of four-and-a-half years, so quite a long time.

It was tough for us, James and me, as a couple and especially on me individually. Believe me; I grieved. I grieved for every single one of those babies. And I must admit that, at some point, I thought I should let James leave so he could meet somebody else, somebody younger who could give him what he wanted. I did not tell him that, but I thought about it quite a lot, especially going into our fourth year of trying. We argued a lot; there was a lot of tension, but somehow through this whole process, we also started to understand and support each other more, I suppose. How did we make it through this time? James is very patient and understanding; he was the rock during these years.

In my interviews, I had quite a few ladies share that they felt distant from their husbands when they miscarried. The women wanted to pour their hearts out, but their partners downplayed what happened.

I totally understand! Because of our experience, I've truly come to understand the fundamental difference between women and men: men want to fix situations whereas women ultimately just need to be heard. For many years, I would avoid talking things through with James because, deep down, I never felt listened to. In the past, when I wanted to share something, I could almost hear his mind searching for a solution to the "problem." And this just frustrated me. After all, this wasn't simply a situation that could be "fixed." He didn't mean to frustrate me; he was simply doing his best with the tools he had. But, nevertheless, the resulting despondency ensued.

I had no one with whom I felt I could share my deepest feelings with, so I felt the only option I had was counseling. I threw myself into being counseled so I could offload to a stranger and walk away feeling I had been listened to without feeling guilty. After a few months, I realized that I did not feel more at ease with my feelings, and eventually, I began to open up to James. I explained to him what I wanted from him. And I was very clear and blunt because not everyone picks up on subtle hints—and he certainly does not. I asked him to just listen to me and to support me. And he did. I am so glad I did that, because he followed my lead and listened, and over time, I could share more and more with him. And he, in turn, albeit carefully, also opened up about his feelings. This enabled me to see the situation from the perspective of the "other person on this journey," too. And I must admit, I had made this journey all about me up to this point.

Did James ever pour his heart out to you as well?

He did, but not until our beautiful baby was born. Since J.J.'s birth, James has often commented that there were times that he felt angry and hopeless at the unfairness of our situation. And he admits that he'd watered down his feelings because he felt he needed to be strong for "us" (somewhere I was clearly failing). In hindsight, I think that it would have been better for me if he had been brutally honest about his feelings. After all, they only echoed my own, and I think hearing it from him would have made it easier for me, to know he was feeling the same way. I think I would have felt less bad about my negative thoughts.

Today, I feel we are strong enough to take whatever challenge life throws at us. It's like we have faced the long battle side-by-side and have been fortunate in our victory. I feel confident enough to confide my deepest feelings to James, and he now shares his thoughts and feelings with me more as well. He seems more at ease with life and shows great empathy toward me and others when they face challenges. He is more loving and affectionate and expresses himself more freely. We both know and understand the highs, lows, and heartache of the fertility journey, and because of this, we not only feel blessed to have the gift of our son, but we appreciate each other so much more. In fact, in two months' time, we shall be exchanging our vows on the beach along the Indian Ocean, our happily ever after!

Congratulations, that is wonderful! Any more advice for couples who are in the midst of their journey?

Keep talking and sharing. It's not easy at first, but you'll be amazed at how a problem shared really is a problem halved because just knowing that your partner is feeling the same way makes it easier to bear—even if your perspectives are different, you'll have understanding. Stand strong together and have lots of cuddles!

Did you ever find out why you miscarried so often?

It turned out that I had moderate endometriosis, and they found some scarring on my fallopian tubes, but the tubes were not blocked. There was always the risk of implantation in my fallopian tubes, which is called an ectopic pregnancy, but there was no concern that I could not get pregnant because of the moderate endometriosis. At some point, I was diagnosed with Graves' disease, which is an autoimmune disease that primarily affects the thyroid and causes hyperthyroidism. But I was able to heal myself from Graves' naturally and without any surgery or medication.

At some point, we also looked into fertility treatments, but as it turned out, these procedures were not available to us. Usually women over 35 who try for at least one year to get pregnant naturally and are labeled with "unexplained infertility" can then go to fertility clinics that are part of the National Health System here in Great Britain. For them, certain procedures are covered by their insurance. We were denied because I already had a daughter and, thus, had "proven" to be able to have a child. We were not entitled to cost-covered IVF in our country. Honestly, though, I was not that disappointed because I preferred to look into natural options before doing something so drastic.

So, looking back at these years, it seems that this was more of a spiritual journey for both James and I than something physically wrong with my body or his. Maybe I had not fully been ready yet or was not in the right place of mind—maybe James had not been either. Either way, it was certainly a time of intense spiritual growth. And it was a lesson—a lesson to trust in my body and to have confidence that my body really knew what to do.

You did not have that confidence before?

No, I did not. So, I focused a lot of my energy on healing my body and making it strong. I changed my diet, I reduced stress, I went to see an acupuncturist, and I made significant lifestyle changes. But there was still a part missing, and that missing puzzle piece was Russell Davis, whom I started working with in the fifth year of our journey. When I first heard of him, I already had done a lot of things that affected me physically, but I had not really addressed my mind.

I started working with Russell in March of 2014 and found out that I was pregnant in July, so just a few months later. It was my sixth pregnancy, and immediately it felt different. After the first miscarriage, I no longer allowed myself to feel excited whenever I got pregnant. I felt the dread of things possibly going wrong throughout the subsequent four pregnancies that all ended up aborting. This time, my sixth pregnancy, I felt elated and full of joy, and I felt completely happy and content and reassured that things would be fine. And I felt that, even if things would not be fine with the pregnancy, I'd still be fine as me, Leah. Does that make sense?

That is a remarkable shift you went through. How did the sessions with Russell work?

He uses hypnotherapy during the session and puts you in a trance. So, I don't remember much about the words that we exchanged, but I do remember leaving the sessions feeling that I had let go of tension and fear that I'd been holding on to. I felt completely at ease with everything afterwards. Russell taught me to understand that our thoughts are just our thoughts and not who we are or what's happening. Our thoughts are based on what has happened in the past, and they are projections of what could happen in the future. Russell taught me to be in the present and reminded me that I have no control over the future—and that I'd be okay no matter what happened.

That was a big awakening for me, and James noticed the changes in me almost immediately. He, too, benefitted from my work with Russell because we talked about it at home, and I also shared all the books that Russell recommended. So, James also experienced a positive effect for himself and us as a couple. We started to communicate much better; we became less frustrated with each other and more understanding. We both carried these changes through to today.

Please help me pinpoint something: You endured a lot—losing five babies, risking your relationship—to have a child. And then you went to a different place in your mind, and you accepted that, even if it would not

happen, you'd still be fine. Was there a pivotal moment that changed things so drastically?

Before working with Russell, I felt that having a baby was the key to my happiness. This was the key to my life; this is what I felt I deserved and I wanted. My happiness was tied to a future child and not to my present. I remember one conversation in particular that was a breakthrough point for me. Russell asked me, "What does having a baby mean to you?" I answered, "It would make me happy; I would feel complete." "What's happiness to you?" he continued. "Just feeling content." "What's feeling content?" he pressed. And I remember getting really angry with him. I felt like he was challenging me to prove that I deserved this child because I wanted it for the right reasons and not because I wanted a child to keep my man or get out of a job or please my parents or whatever. But, actually, what he was trying to do was help me see if the thoughts and feelings that I'd put behind having a baby were the truth or just something I fantasized about.

So, when he asked, "How would you feel if you had a baby?" and I answered, "I would feel happy and complete," he tried to help me understand that I could feel happy and complete now, in my current life, regardless of what my circumstances were. That was a turning point for me because I realized that I had not had a baby in my arms for eighteen years, and I was still fine and fairly happy and content in my life. I've got a lot of children around me—I work with children—and I can still feel that love. I still feel blessed with the things I do have, like my health, my partner, my daughter, all of those things. I have reason to feel grateful and blessed. Our sessions helped me see that.

But there was also the fear factor behind me wanting to have a child so badly. It's the fear of the unknown. And with Russell's help, I could see myself in the unknown and still be okay. When you are there—in the unknown—it's actually not as bad as you think it will be, and life still goes on. You can still be happy and enjoy life.

Please explain: what was the "fear of the unknown" for you? Let's go deep now.

Yes, and that's fine. I had this deep fear that James would resent me one day because I had not been able to give him what he wanted. Even if he would not show this, I would know it; I would feel it. That was one of my biggest fears. After this particular conversation with Russell, I understood: what will be will be. If James would really resent me, we could talk about it and decide what to do then, whether that was ten years from now or two years or whenever. Even if he would have decided to leave, I'd be okay.

Sure, I would have been sad that the relationship came to an end and that things had not worked out the way we had hoped, but I'd still be okay. It would have been a darker part of my life, but still a part where I could choose to see the positive aspects. One positive I would have seen would have been that James could now go and get what he wanted and that I loved him enough to allow that—that he could meet somebody else and have what he wanted. There is always a lesson in the painful parts of our lives that can help us to grow on our journey.

Thank you very much for your honesty and depth. I really enjoyed talking to you.

Now I would like to tell you that I think it's very good and important that you are writing this book.

I appreciate that; thank you. Why would you say so?

Because you are sharing our different perspectives on fertility, in particular, and health, in general. I now know that there are a lot of health issues that are connected to mindset, and by changing our mindset, we can increase our health. The medical community, however, is usually not open to taking into consideration methods of healing that don't follow the scientific textbook. That's how they are trained—it's really not their fault. But as a result, people often have no idea about all the things they can do themselves to cure diseases and get better or, as in our case, become more fertile.

As I mentioned, I was diagnosed with Graves' disease by my endocrinologist. When I went back to see him nine months later, he expected me to be worse and that I would have to have my thyroid taken out. He was stunned to see that I was in remission, and he could not understand how that had happened. I told him how I had changed my life, reduced stress, leveled up my diet, and that I had a different mindset now. He was dismissive of it all and just said, "Oh, no, you are just lucky." This smart and nice man could not even fathom that there are other methods of healing out there than the ones he was trained in. So, he had to dismiss my success as a fluke.

That's a problem. People who want to get better are under the impression that their path to health can only go through medical intervention. But there is a lot of work women can do on their minds and their bodies in order to increase their chances to conceive. I, myself, became a fertility reflexologist after my journey, and I see firsthand what positive effect this type of work has on my patients. Once more and more people get this message, there will be change for the better, and we won't have to go through so much heartache, not just with fertility but with health in general. I healed my Graves' disease and went on to have a healthy pregnancy and a healthy child. And if our interview helps even one couple conceive, I'll be elated!

CHAPTER 5

Jenny

"The dark night of the soul." For Jennifer, this is not just an expression; it was a brutal reality. The darkest days of her journey toward motherhood were spent in a mental health facility on an island off the coast of England. This journalist-turned-acupuncturist was hospitalized after spiraling out of control and becoming suicidal because she so desperately wished for a family. After six weeks of treatment, soul searching, and regaining her footing, Jenny left the hospital with the first inkling that, even if she did not have children, she would be okay. She says, "I had been through something so bad and came out alive, so I knew I could survive anything else that life threw at me. I would be okay no matter what." Today, she's not just okay, but considers herself "the luckiest woman alive."

A mutual journalist friend introduced us, and we immediately found common ground: we had both started our career in journalism, and while I left Austria to report from New York, Jenny had left her native Boston to report from London, a city where she still resides. As a print and eventual TV journalist, Jenny covered politics and foreign affairs, which meant that, for over fifteen years, she traveled all over the globe to interview world leaders and dignitaries. She loved her work, even if it meant long hours, lots of pressure, and dating men who thrived on thrills.

"I was drawn to the men in my field, most of them foreign correspondents, who were adrenalin junkies themselves," Jenny remembered, and I could see why men were attracted to this smart and beautiful woman with her long blonde hair and blue eyes. "I did have the baby conversation from time to time with men I was in serious relationships with, but it was hard to get a commitment if the other person just wanted to rush to Iraq or Afghanistan to cover another insurgency." Jenny realized that, if she wanted to get serious about having a family, she needed to make a drastic shift. So, when she was around 38, she completely changed her social life and stopped hanging out in the clubs her colleagues went to. She also left the world of current affairs and started to train to become an acupuncturist—all of which would ultimately lead her to motherhood at 42 and another baby at 45.

Jenny: At first, things went well. I celebrated my 40th birthday, and I was very happy. I was thinking everything would be fine; I would meet the man of my dreams, etc. I had ups and downs, but overall, I wasn't panicking. However, my 41st birthday hit me really hard. I still hadn't met the man I wanted to marry and have children with. And soon after, I went into total, flat-out panic. I absolutely, totally freaked out.

I started to think that I was losing my fertility because my periods changed. They now came every twenty-four days instead of longer, and they were much shorter and lighter. So, I thought, my God, I am perimenopausal. Anyway, that part was not true, as I went to see an acupuncturist, and she helped me boost my periods, and they became stronger again. But I had already started to seriously doubt my fertility. So, I went to a fertility specialist and inquired about freezing my eggs. Without even doing one test on me, she said "No, you are too old; the quality of your eggs would not be good enough." That was a major blow.

As a next step, I put my name on a list for donor sperm. I was told I had to wait nine months to a year because there was a shortage. By then, seven years ago, the rules had changed in Great Britain around sperm donation. Previously, donations had been anonymous, but that had led to many children growing up without having any way to find out about their fathers. There were all sorts of issues surrounding identity and that sort of thing, so they changed the rules.

The donors were no longer anonymous, but as a result, there were a lot less men willing to give their sperm.

I still went through the process, but shortly before my 42nd birthday, I was in yet another disastrous relationship, and this time, it sent me over the edge. Something clicked inside me, and I thought, that's it; I've lost my opportunity to have a family. I had been depressed before—in fact, depression runs deep in my family—but this time I spiraled into the worst depression of my life. I became unbearably anxious and thought that I'd lost my fertility. I thought I was never going to have the family that I longed for. I thought that it was over for me. I became absolutely desperate and fell apart. I became suicidal.

Bettina: That sounds horrifying. Please help me understand: what exactly was it that you longed for so deeply—the connection with another human being?

Yes, it was the longing for a family unit, the longing for a husband, a decent, wonderful man in my life, and a family, a child. I was so lonely; I could not bear it any longer. I spun out into a million different pieces. When I saw my psychiatrist for a session, she said, "Jenny, you are very, very ill. I am committing you to a residential care facility." I ended up in a hospital for six weeks.

But before I was admitted, I did something that I think is really important to mention for your book. Before I went into the hospital, I decided that I needed to be with the child I so often fantasized about. I needed to birth this fantasy child of mine. I remember I went into my bedroom, turned off all the lights, and lit candles. I got undressed and kind of envisioned going into labor and birthing this child of mine, my daughter. I remember squatting on the floor, pretending to give birth to this beautiful girl, whom I then picked up and put to my breast. I sat with her for about an hour and held her like that. Then I wrapped this fantasy child into a blanket, and I went into my back garden. And I remember throwing her into the air and saying to God, "If you're going to bring her back, I am ready; I am waiting for her!" I had tears streaming down my face because I didn't know whether I was going to have this precious daughter that I so longed for.

What a beautiful story! This could be interpreted as either a wonderful, heroic tale of a woman's courage or the display of a psychotic episode. Which one is it for you?

I did not feel crazy when I went through this. In fact, it was a very conscious choice to birth this fantasy child that I somehow felt around me. In hindsight, I believe two things: I believe I called in her spirit and gave her to God to potentially give back to me. I think I was communicating with God to please hurry up, because I was ready and waiting. Second, I think I was so desperate that it was a way of taking back some sort of control in my life. I had felt so powerless, but by acting out giving this spirit to God, I was able to retake control of the situation. I was doing *something* instead of just lying there on my bed day after day, longing and feeling insane. So, birthing my daughter felt right, and it felt good, yet it was not enough to prevent me from becoming very ill and being hospitalized.

I cannot help but wonder if what you did, giving birth to your fantasy daughter, is a powerful example of women's wisdom—of something bigger and ancient and more instinctual than we can grasp with our minds today. Thank you for sharing so openly.

I thought, if we do this interview, let's do it full-on. As I mentioned, I still had to go to the clinic, which was on an island off the coast of England. I would go for long walks and just sort of talk to this daughter that I had imagined, as if her spirit was flying around me. I kept the connection alive and strong, which was good for my soul. Oh, I forgot to mention that I had a fertility test done before I checked into the clinic. And one day the psychiatrist in the residential hospital asked if I would like to know the results. I said, "Yes, I should know." He said, "Your fertility is fine. You are a 42-year-old woman, and you can have a baby, and there's nothing stopping you from having a baby." And, even though he was my psychiatrist and I was still under medication, he said to me, "I also know that you're going to get married and have a baby." "How do you know?" I asked him. "I don't know how, but I do know."

This man and this time at the clinic lifted my spirits, and I started to feel sane again. I now know I had reasonably good fertility for my age, but I also had something even more valuable: when I got out of the clinic, I had the first inkling that, even if I did not have children, I would survive. I knew that I'd been through the worst of it now and that I was never going to be that desperate again. I knew I could survive anything else that life threw at me.

I left the clinic in September, and by the year's end, I had met two men. One lived in London, where I live, and the other one in Boston, where I am from. In January, I went off to a yoga retreat in India, and I wondered if I should really start seeing somebody who lived so far away. Even though I was American and was a bit drawn to the man in Boston, I made the sensible choice and called the man in London back after my return. I am so grateful I did. We went on a second date. He invited me to his birthday party, and shortly after, we got together. I was very open with him about the depression and that I needed to take pills every day. I am still on medication, by the way, and was through my pregnancies. It's important I take my pills since I am now responsible for little ones as well, not just myself. Maybe one day I can get off them, but not yet.

Anyway, I told him about my hospitalization, and he did not seem particularly fazed by it. After maybe a couple of months, *he* actually brought up the baby talk. Thomas was 47 at that time, and I was 42. He said "Look, I know we don't know each other very well, but should we start trying for a baby while we are getting to know each other better? Because it can take us a year or so anyway to conceive, right?" I thought, I really like this guy, and I agreed it wouldn't happen very quickly, so I figured it was a good idea and we should try. Month one, nothing. Month two, I was pregnant.

You and Thomas were together for four months when you got pregnant? For real?

Yeah, it was pretty insane, but I felt very calm and excited, especially once I found out that I was going to have a daughter! I was like, "Oh, my god, this is my daughter, the one I sent to God, and she came back to me." It was the most incredible manifestation of my life. It still makes me so happy to think back on that day.

I did have challenges, though. I was sick up to eight times every single day for the first six months of my pregnancy. That part was really a shock to the system, as I had seen myself as an earth mama, barefoot and floating around in a caftan. I thought I'd have an easy pregnancy. Not so. I was terribly sick, and it was really draining.

Thomas had asked me to marry him two weeks after we found out I was pregnant. (He swears that he had already planned to ask me anyway.) I was more than happy to marry him, but because the pregnancy was so tough, mentally and physically, we postponed it until the following year when our daughter was six months old. The funny thing is, we got a really good deal because the Church of England has this special rate: if you buy a wedding, you can get a christening thrown in for free *(laughs)*.

Potentially, there is a big difference between having the fantasy of starting a family and then living the reality of meeting your man and having a child within one year. How did you deal with the new reality?

It was not an easy first year because I felt so terrible, and I did not anticipate how much change and turmoil this new life would bring. From the moment I met Thomas, there was something in my soul that whispered, "This is the right man," but I did not really know him yet. It took time, and gradually, I learned who he was, and I learned that my soul had been absolutely right—that he was wise and kind, good and sensitive, and caring and supportive. He saw me through a very difficult pregnancy, all while we looked for a new home, prepared for the arrival of Arizona, and planned a wedding.

We had lots and lots of changes within a short period of time. It became clearer and clearer, though, that I was the luckiest woman on earth. We took our daughter on our honeymoon to the Middle East, where I had worked before as a journalist. We went to Turkey and Lebanon and Syria before the war, and we trekked through the countries with our daughter in the backpack. And I thought, "Yeah, this is all I ever wanted."

I am so happy for you to have this new life now. You were 42 when your daughter was born, and your son arrived two weeks shy of your 45th birthday. What have you learned about yourself as a mom in her 40s and about having children later in life?

I honestly think that having a child later on is the best idea anybody could ever have. Speaking for myself, I was able to achieve so much of what I wanted to, and so I came to motherhood feeling like I knew myself pretty well. I think I am much calmer now than I would have been when I was younger. I am more centered and not so easily rattled by the demands of being a mom or by my kids' needs or temper tantrums—nor am I very influenced by the opinion of other adults. Not much fazes me. I know how to take care of myself, which helps me take better care of my children.

I love motherhood in my 40s, but it's hard to advise women to wait because it's awful to think that some people might not be able to get pregnant. I once heard a fertility expert say, "The idea of fertility dropping off a cliff at 40 is faulty because someone can have poor fertility at 25, and she's also going to have poor fertility at 40. Or, someone can have pretty good fertility and that carries on through life and into her late 40s, when she transitions from perimenopause to menopause."

It's very hard to advise, but I think those who do have children later in life are very blessed—the parents as well as the children.

CHAPTER 6

Ellen

When I first heard about Ellen, I became rather excited. A natural and healthy pregnancy at 46? Now there was a woman I was dying to interview. Ellen came highly recommended by a mutual friend of ours, an emergency room doctor in New York City, who turned to Ellen whenever she was in need of holistic healing herself. As a holistic health practitioner, Ellen was also trained in craniosacral osteopathy (an alternative medicine intended to relieve pain and tension by gentle manipulations of the skull) and in family constellation (also an alternative, therapeutic method of discovering a person's underlying family bonds and forces that have been carried unconsciously over several generations). In less fancy wording, Ellen is a "natural healer."

When we met on Skype, I found a woman as salt of the earth as they come. Her short brown hair framed her oval face, and her whole demeanor seemed to be wide open toward me and our agenda at hand. As may be the case for many modern-day healers, Ellen's life was neither easy nor a straight road—she was born in Communist East Germany before ultimately living and working in the United States. In our interview, Ellen dug deep to share her life's path and wisdom with me. To understand her journey toward motherhood, we went way back in time.

Ellen: Before I turned 30, I never had a period, not even once. I went to doctors for tests and exams, but none of them could give me a reason. I always had too little estrogen and too much testosterone. And when I asked the doctors for a reason for my condition, they would shake their heads and say, "That's just what it is. Some women have more testosterone; others don't." They diagnosed me with PCOS, and I never received an answer from academic medicine as to why I had never gotten my period and, subsequently, could not become a mother—something which I'd desired from very early in life. This made me deeply sad. I started to speak to my unborn baby, saying things like, "Sorry, my child, we may meet in another life, not this one." I was truly missing the baby that I was told I could never have.

When I turned 30, something life-changing happened. I decided to see a holistic health practitioner in the town I lived in to get to the bottom of my fertility issue. We had six very intense sessions, where she would work with me on a mental, physical, and emotional level. The emotional level was significant because, at this point, I was working as a physical therapist, and I noticed that, for some patients, when we healed one part of their body, a little later the pain would come back in another spot. There was an underlying hurt that kept showing up in different locations.

It was right before our last session that I uncovered the reason for my missing period. I was at home one night when, suddenly, I remembered a memory that I had suppressed for decades. In my mind, I saw myself back in my parents' apartment as a 6-year-old girl, standing by the window, when all of a sudden, a young child, maybe two or three years old, fell to her death from the window above.

I was in shock, but what happened next paralyzed me. When her mother realized what had happened, she rushed down and threw herself over her little daughter and cried. She cried so loud, with so much pain and heartbreak, that it went right through me. She cried like a wounded wolf. This mother made the most horrific and gut-wrenching sounds I have ever heard a human being make. To say it was terrible is not enough to describe it. And in that moment, I realized that this could be me. One day, I could be this mother who loses her child. And it could be me who experiences this unimaginable hurt and pain.

The suffering of this mother really got to me. It still does. I get chills just speaking of it, four decades later.

Bettina: My God, me too. I am holding back tears.

At this moment, as a six-year-old girl, I decided to never have a child because this could happen to me. Now, today, I know from my work that the decisions of your mind can significantly impact your body. I know that my body heard me and understood me, and the hormonal system did everything it could to fulfill my wish. Too much testosterone was the way to ensure I would never be a mother. After this revelation and my sixth and final session with the holistic health practitioner, my period came for the first time in my adult life. I remember it clearly. I bought a bottle of wine and called my mother—we were both so happy. And I have had my period at regular intervals, like clockwork, ever since.

That is an incredible and really moving story. Thank you for being so open to sharing it. Now I am wondering, why did it take another sixteen years for you to conceive the child you were longing for?

After this experience, I became a holistic health counsellor myself, as physical therapy was not enough anymore—I wanted to really go deep in my work. But I still had issues that I needed to resolve for myself and experiences I needed to have. I had dear friends who would say things like, "Oh, poor Ellen, she would so much desire a husband and a child." But, on the inside, I felt somewhat different, or at least I lived a life at odds with these desires.

During the day, I established myself with my healing work, but at night I lived a life that was not conducive in the least to meeting a loving man. I was emotionally confused and did not know who I really was. Was I the good woman? The wild one? The whore or the housewife? The mother or the sinner? It was a tough time for me, and true to form, I usually attracted men who did not want a family, or at least not anymore, because they'd had children who had died at a young age. I was also in love with a man for fifteen years. Even though we were not a couple anymore, he was the one I wanted. We made love whenever we met. For him it was sex, but these hours meant the world to me. And, so, the years went by.

In the spring of 2003, I "woke up." I needed to put an end to all these years of heartbreak. I wrote him a letter and broke it off. I let go and opened up to a new man. I visualized him, wrote about him in my journal, and invited him into my life. At 36 years old, I met my husband, Ralf, who is seven years my senior. I knew from the day I met him that I would be with him, and I saw us both leaving Germany and moving to the United States together, which was a huge leap. I didn't even speak English at the time because it had been mandatory to learn Russian when I was growing up. But that's what I intuitively felt.

I was also very frank and open with him about my past, my partners, and my infertility. For even though I had my period now, I had not gotten pregnant for years, despite not using contraceptives. My infertility was fine with him because he, too, did not want to have children anymore. Ralf had lost his own little girl when she was just 14 years old. Imagine that! But this was the man I was drawn to and for whom I completely changed my life. Ralf is the first relationship I ever had where I stayed faithful and committed—it's the only relationship I've been in for the long haul. By the time I met Ralf, I really wanted a man . . . and I wanted a child. We both had a lot of work ahead of us.

You found the love of your life, but he was done having children. If I didn't know the ending, I would say that this is a rather tragic story. What did you do?

Well, I had been in contact with my child sixteen years before I actually conceived her. That may sound strange or unusual for many people, but I believe that there is communication between a mother or father and the spirit of a child long before the child is conceived. And I would tell Ralf from time to time that I was communicating with our child and that we should invite the soul to come and live with us if it wanted to.

But Ralf did not want to hear any of it, and he and I we were so good together, we loved and supported each other so much, that I stopped talking to him about it. Yet, I still kept the window open for my desire to welcome in a child. At the same time, I was very aware that I had to work through my own deep-seated fears: the fear that my child may die before me and the fear that I would be all alone in my old age.

In 2004, we moved to New York City, and I got lucky and established my business quickly through the help of new friends. Three years later, my mother, whom I was very close to, died. When she passed, she said to me, "Ellen, I strongly feel that you will have a child one day." And, indeed, a year later, I fell pregnant. It was a most difficult time for us because the recession hit us hard in 2008, and we were having financial troubles.

When I told Ralf that I was pregnant, he was devastated. He cried, his blood pressure shot up, and he was desperate and beside himself. It was not the right time, not the right place to bring in a new life. When I realized that he was not able to deal with the pregnancy and could not manage all the fears that were coming up for him, I looked at the situation soberly. I thought, this man will stay with me until the end—a child will leave me again. In this moment, at this time, I chose my husband over my unborn child.

Pardon? You had an abortion?

No, I could not do that. But I went into the bathroom, and I caressed my belly, and I whispered, "If it's possible for you, can you please go and find other parents? Daddy just cannot do it right now." An abortion was not an option, but the natural way was okay with me. Days later, I had the miscarriage. And I celebrated my miscarriage; I really did. I had candles in the room and soft music, and I consciously experienced what was happening. I can deal with crisis situations really well, so I was able to stay open and present and to feel the connection to all the other women who had miscarried before.

It was like a gift for me to now understand what others had gone through. And I felt so lucky and content that I had known what it meant to be pregnant, even if only for a short time. What a feeling of happiness that was! Sure, I cried and was sad, but afterwards I grew again. I began to see the miscarriage as an enrichment of my life. And, for Ralf, he was also very sad and relieved at the same time.

Do you, indeed, think that you made the miscarriage happen?

It was really an invitation to the soul to leave if possible, so I invited the miscarriage, rather than making it happen. But if the child would have been determined to be born, this would not have worked. Ralf and I believe that it was the soul of our Rose that wanted to come all those years ago. But it was okay for her to return at a later time; she was good with that. She likes it better now.

The other point is, I had made my choice, and I had chosen my husband. I had made peace with losing the pregnancy if it should happen. So, I miscarried at age 41, and we continued our lives. We both felt we needed to be closer to nature and moved to Maine, where we now live in the woods close to the ocean. We found our footing again and did not use contraception when we made love. When I turned 45 and did not get pregnant again, I was like, "Okay, that's it; I am too old now. It's over." But I still talked to the boy child I saw from time to time sitting at our kitchen table. I kept the connection alive and, at the same time, felt the pain of having lost this option.

I was sad that I would not experience motherhood this time and that I would be alone when I was old and dying, which was still a deep fear of mine. I had to make peace to find peace. I had a wonderful husband, clients in the United States and in Europe, and I had other people's children in my life. I thought, "I have so much; I just cannot have everything, and that's okay."

On New Year's Eve, 2012, I performed a ritual in which I deeply and wholeheartedly let go of my fears of losing a child before me and, more important, of dying alone. The process was simple: I lit up some sage, wrote it all on a piece of paper, and burned the paper in the sage. But this was not just a ritual; there was real power behind it. I was centered, focused, and intense. I really meant it and went very deep. I came out on the other end with a sense of total freedom, of being liberated from the fears.

And then it happened?

In May 2013, I felt it like lightning. It happened. When the doctor confirmed my pregnancy, I cried and cried. What if I would miscarry again? What if Ralf could not handle it again? But Ralf was excited, even though he was concerned about our age, as I was already 46 and he was 53. But I said, "If a child comes so late to us, the child wants to stay."

I did not do any tests or see the doctor again until my second trimester. And I enjoyed my pregnancy immensely. My skin was beautiful, my belly small and gorgeous, and I looked wonderful and glowing. By then I had been eating macrobiotic foods for twenty years and did not feel the need for any testing other than measuring the belly and listening to the heartbeat. I knew that my boy, who turned out to be a girl, was healthy. But I stopped working four months before the due date, as I did not want to hear about my clients; I just wanted to go inside and be with my child.

Naturally, I planned a home birth, and that's how it started out, with my water breaking at home. But then my labor stopped, and we drove to the hospital in a snowstorm. I refused the epidural and any other medication, and I pushed through the pain. I pushed like an animal, and again, I felt so connected to all the women before me. This gave me such strength and endurance. Isn't it amazing to give birth? It was incredible!

Yes. My birth was also natural and the most empowering experience of my life!

They put Rose on my breast right after birth, and I have been breastfeeding her ever since *(laughs)*. I decided not to return to work for three years because I wanted to be with her. Although I may not have as many years with her as a younger mother might, it will probably work out to more hours in the end because I was with her during this critical time. It was my conscious choice to lay a loving, solid foundation for her for the rest of her life, and so we've spent every single day together since she was born. Ralf works from home, so he is around too. By the way, the man thanks me every single day for having believed and birthed this child. He could not be happier.

And we decided to live longer now that we have this young child. Through the many experiences in my professional career, I've come to believe that we can influence our health and longevity, and Ralf and I have adapted our mindset in addition to living a very healthy lifestyle. I no longer fear that I will die too young. I am shooting for late 80s or beyond. On the other hand, do I sometimes feel old? Am I tired right now? You bet! Childcare is more demanding than work. But maybe you know the saying: with little children, the days are long, and the years are short. I look forward to her starting Waldorf kindergarten, but I would not have had it any other way. I have loved being with her and nurturing her daily.

You now work with women who desire motherhood. Any parting wisdom you'd like to share with us?

Every woman struggling with fertility should hear one thing: you are *fertile*! When, in my 20s, I heard a doctor tell me that I was not fertile, it did something to me. It changed me. How do you remedy that? I reach women through bodywork and the conversations we have while I touch them. Fertility means not only birthing children but also baking cakes, writing stories, or planting a garden. Let's go from there.

I myself believe that, in the sixteen years between my first period and Rose's conception, I was indeed fertile, but my fertility was covered by stuff, like me not making a commitment; me being fearful of losing a child; me not making room for a baby in my lifestyle, etc. My fertility was covered, and I had to first work out and heal the different aspects of my life. I encourage my patients to make room by "making yourself empty." And by always, always keeping the connection to the soul of your child alive. Leave your heart open for a child—regardless of what the circumstances are right now!

CHAPTER 7

MIND Action Steps

Choose to Become a Fertility Rebel in Your Own Right

For the sake of all the unborn children who want to come into this world through our bodies and into our loving arms, let's step out of the cultural norm and shake up some common beliefs that do not serve us. Let's refuse to buy into the collective dogma—become a fertility rebel, if you will. When I say "rebel," I don't mean the adolescent rebel, one who pushes against authority with an *I will show you* attitude. Don't get me wrong; this type of approach can be advantageous, but it won't serve you here. *I will prove you wrong* is too narrow a view and too tight of an energy to hold for mothers-to-be.

We want expansion, not constriction. We want joy on our paths, not portents of grimness and gloom. The fertility rebel I am talking about is the empowered, mature woman, one who chooses to make up her own mind and has the courage to go against mainstream opinions and judgments. So, collect all the information you feel you need and then check in with yourself as to what is true for you and what is not. Make peace with the information/judgment/opinion that does not work for you and let it go. You don't need approval to choose what's right. You march to the beat of your own drum, writing your own rules instead of having authorities do it for you.

Don't Give Your Power over to the Person with the Most Certainty

People will come up with statistics and their own reasoning for what's right or wrong, but we must never allow the person with the most certainty (usually a doctor or other authoritative figure) to win out over our own inner wisdom, especially when it comes to such delicate matters as creating new life and guiding your children into adulthood. We all need to check in with ourselves. If your gut tells you something, listen. I am not saying you should discount someone because he or she is a doctor. I am, however, suggesting that you do not blindly believe someone just because this person is a doctor. If you instinctively, or by research, feel that the information you are given does not apply, trust yourself.

Step away from the Stats Buffet

Practice mental hygiene and stop consuming information that's "dirty" and leaves you feeling bad. Next time you read the paper or watch the news on TV, I want you to pay close attention to how you feel before you see a story about the atrocities of war, the shooting of kids in their school, or the dangers and risks of birthing a severely handicapped child after 40, and how you feel after. Has your mood dropped? Do you feel the tightness in your body? Are your shoulders slumped, your mouth tense?

Words and pictures have an immediate effect on all of us physically. For the time being—and for all the time between now and the birth of your child—I advise you to step away from the fertility stats buffet and stop reading about all the things that can go wrong with your body and your child. Be informed and know your rights, but don't dwell on things. Walk away when you have all the information you need. I repeat: step away from the negativity buffet.

Realize That You Are Not a Statistic

When I was pregnant, I shrugged off all the statistics anybody would put in front of me. I figured that, just because I was a certain age, I'd be lumped into a statistic with all women who had not taken care of their bodies the way I had, who had diseases I did not, who were possibly mentally unbalanced or in unsupportive relationships, or had a long line of disorders running through their family history, which had absolutely nothing to do with me and my health and my chances and my risks. Whatever their reasons were for not conceiving or miscarrying or birthing babies that were not optimally healthy, their reasons were not mine. I would have my own reasons (or not), thank you very much.

Defining women by a statistic does not make sense to me. You are not a statistic, and you are much more than a number, more than the sum of your age or your FSH or your egg quality, because these numbers can be significantly improved with the right holistic regimen. Stop believing in absolutes. And, as Julia Indichova, author of *Inconceivable* and first-time mom at 42 puts it so beautifully, "Dare to have an opinion that defies the certainty of studies and statistics!"

Practice Radical Self-Love

A woman who loves herself, who respects and honors her body, can be the best mother any child could dream of because she has a vast reserve of love and strength she can dip into. Let me quote Chinese medicine expert Andrew Loosely, who, for decades, has helped women realize their dream for a baby: "Is the amount of love you're allowed to give to yourself dependent on that positive pregnancy test?" If so, we really need to change that.

Now, before conception, is the time to fall madly and deeply in love with yourself and to fill up potentially empty tanks. Please don't go into the journey with the fear or expectation that something could be broken with you. And if you find out that there are challenges, drench—not dip—yourself in self-love! Here are a few tips on how to do that:

1) Create a gratitude jar. Dedicate a beautiful glass jar or container and, every day, put in a piece of paper on which you have listed three things you are grateful for (about yourself as well as your life in general). Find three new things every day and do this for thirty days. Rinse and repeat.

2) Do something you love to do and that brings you joy. Do you like to take pictures? Reach for your camera and click away. Do you like to cook? Spend time in your kitchen. To run? Grab your shoes and head out the door.

3) Meet with friends face-to-face. When women who share a close bond get together, they release the love hormone, oxytocin. We are way beyond the years when gossip dominated the conversation—it's all about depth and honesty now—and you should get a hit of oxytocin whenever you can.

4) Love your body. Create little rituals—for example, after a shower, take extra time to moisturize your legs, arms, or any part of the body you are especially fond of. Start to think of your body as the future home of your child.

Watch Your Language and Lovingly Reframe

Start paying attention to the self-talk that is constantly going on in your beautiful head. How do you speak to yourself when nobody else is listening? What are you telling yourself that's not conducive to your wish to conceive and nurture a child? Switch out the self-punishing talk with more loving perspectives:

- I am the perfect age to become the best mother to my child.
- Every woman's path in life is different and divinely guided.
- I did nothing wrong. I am where I am supposed to be.
- I was guided to where I am today. This is my path, and I embrace it.
- My body is vibrant and fertile.
- I have time to improve my health and optimize my chances to conceive.
- I can work out any kinks in the system in the months to come.
- I know it's all about the quality of my eggs, not the quantity of my egg reserve.
- My egg quality will improve with the right regimen.
- My body is strong and knows how to carry a child to term.
- My body is wise, and it is capable of birthing a baby.

Give Yourself Time

I heard it over and over in my interviews: babies have their own timeline, and if we want to push it and force it, it's not going to work in our favor. When we feel we have not enough time, we tend to panic, which changes our body chemistry. When the body panics, it gets the message that we are not safe, and it's harder to conceive a child when the body is feeling unsafe. Also, if you are not in a good place financially or feel your partner is not quite the right person to have a child with or have similar messages of "I am not safe," give yourself permission to try to find the right man or to figure it out instead of saying, "It's now or never."

It took me a couple of years to work out my own issues of feeling unsafe and to get my relationship on the most solid and unshakable ground, and so I conceived at 43 instead of 40/41. Allow yourself time to work things out. I know that this goes against the "quick, don't waste another month" mentality that's out there, but that's also what the vast majority of the women I interviewed said. If you use extra time wisely and diligently and work your stuff out, time is your friend.

Seek Professional Counseling Now, Not after You've Become a Mother

There are many reasons for wanting a child, all of which should be examined closely and honestly. Do you want somebody who loves you for the next eighteen years? Do you want someone who depends on you so you feel significant? Do you want out of your job and think that pregnancy would be the most appropriate reason for you to quit? Do you want a child because you still don't know what to do with your life or career and this would buy you some time? Do you think a child might bring you the happiness you otherwise won't have? Do you feel a child would improve your otherwise shaky relationship? Are you secretly in love with someone else but think that a baby would make you stay with your husband? Do you want a child to make up for your bad childhood?

The desire for a child can significantly multiply when we feel the biological door closing. This often clouds our judgment. I do not need to point out that none of the scenarios above, all real-life examples, will work out well—you will still be the same person with the same issues after you give birth as you were before, just way more stressed and now responsible for a tiny human being who needs you to be the best version of yourself, not the conflicted, wounded version.

You cannot (should not) mother another being if you have not done the necessary soul work to overcome your own issues. My advice is to seek out professional counseling for your mental health, your professional path, or your relationship with your spouse now, before you even try to conceive, in order to really get to the bottom of what drives you toward motherhood. Believe me; you don't want to wake up a mother one day and regret it.

One of the women who openly wrote about her regrets in having a child past 40 is Stacie Krajchir. Check out her article in the *Huffington Post* titled "Fortyhood: Why You're Too Old to Have a Baby After 40." She starts with, "Here's the deal: you always want what you can't have. Before I had my own baby, when I saw someone pushing a stroller down the street, I would hurt—physically—with yearning. Motherhood was the club I so deeply wanted to belong to, and I was determined to become a member by any means necessary." The headline to her story is misleading, as she is talking about her own experience and not others' experiences, but you may find it helpful.

CHAPTER 8

Pillar Two: BODY

Your Health Is Your Fertility

When it comes to life-altering situations, I like to have someone familiar, someone I trust and feel comfortable with by my side. Three months before I conceived my son, I found myself in the 9th district of Vienna, Austria, in a rather familiar setting, amidst antique couches and chairs and underneath a humongous crystal chandelier in the waiting room of my OB/GYN. Even though I had left my birthplace in the mid-90s and lived in the United States ever since, I still continued seeing my doctor twice a year whenever I came back to visit my family. What can I say? I'm a loyal patient.

As I excitedly thumbed through magazines on pregnancy and parenting, I couldn't help but smile. This would be a big surprise for him. As the door to his room swung open, I stormed into his office, plopped down on the chair, and exclaimed, "Doc, I've changed my mind! I do want to have a child!"

I think his jaw would have dropped all the way to the ground if there hadn't been a floor to stop it. He looked at me bewildered and bellowed, "Oh *no*!" so loudly that the receptionist may have heard. I remember cracking up laughing. I had known this man for over twenty years, and his unintentionally inappropriate exclamations are legendary. After all, this was the same man who had delivered my goddaughter Valentina. When he met her again sixteen years later for her first OB/GYN appointment, he jollily said, "Good to see you, Valentina, after all these years. I see you have developed very nicely," precisely as the girl made herself comfortable on the examining chair. Valentina still blushes when she tells the story, but he thought nothing of it.

"That was not the reaction I had actually hoped for," I said, still laughing as the expression on his face quickly changed from mild horror to moderate concern.

"Sorry, I mean, ah," he tried to backpedal, "I mean, oh, no, now we have wasted valuable years!" I remember very distinctly (and so does he) what I did next. I reached over the desk and put my right hand on his forearm. "No worries, Doc," I said in a calm and reassuring voice, "You'll see. Next time I come to your office, I will be pregnant!"

Was that a pie-in-the-sky fantasy of mine? Maybe. Because I was 43 at that time, most people may even think I was delusional to make such a proclamation. But here are the reasons why my doctor chose not to inundate me with scary statistics or take away my hope and conviction: I had just spent two years eradicating my fears around motherhood, putting my relationship on rock solid ground and learning to care for another being (yes, I give our rescue dog, Georgia, big credit for "growing me up"). I had even started a brand-new, fun career in tourism that fulfilled me on many levels. I had joy and excitement again in my life. I ate rather well and cooked healthy meals at home for 80 percent of the time. I was not particularly stressed, nor was I anxious about my age, and my body felt strong and healthy at 152 pounds, despite the fact that I had not seen a gym from the inside in years. Last but not least, my ovaries and uterus looked, according to my doctor, "perfect."

Now, was that enough to guarantee me a pregnancy? No, of course not. We are all wise enough to know that there are absolutely no guarantees in life (other than death). Yet we are also experienced enough to know that, whenever we show up 100 percent prepared for a meeting, arrive well-dressed and confident for a date, or stay calm and collected during an emergency, we set ourselves up for the best-possible positive outcome.

Hope that natural pregnancy at 40+ is possible and the conviction that we can achieve it are the only two attitudes that can carry us over the finish line.

I am grateful for my doctor for not trying to erode my hope, despite the fact that we both knew that my body was not infallible:

- When I was 30 years old, I scheduled an MRI for my recurring headaches. The exam revealed a three- to four-millimeter tumor on my pituitary gland (also known as the master gland of the body). These brain tumors can overproduce a variety of hormones—in my case, prolactin. My tumor was benign at that point in time.
- In my mid to late 30s, I had a fibroid as large as a tennis ball in my uterus. I was taken aback by the size of it, but the fibroid had not caused me any discomfort, and I saw no reason to surgically remove it.
- Also in my late 30s, my doctor found dozens of little cysts on both of my ovaries. This can cause the ovaries to enlarge and, if left untreated, cause infertility. The more common term for this is polycystic ovary syndrome (PCOS), but my doctor never called it that. We agreed that we would monitor it.
- Recently we found out that my thyroid was slightly "underactive." In more severe cases, this is called hypothyroidism, which can cause miscarriages and other complications. So, my doctor put me on a low dosage of medication to help my body get pregnant and keep the pregnancy (expert advice: an in-depth, full-panel thyroid blood test is a *must* before you try to conceive).

Become the CEO of Your Own Health

I am telling you about my body's setbacks because, if you are a woman within the "high risk pregnancy" age range, chances are, you have experienced physical challenges along the journey of your life, too. This is not unusual, and it does *not* necessarily mean that you cannot have a child over 40. What it does mean, though, is that you need to make your health your number one priority.

In my mind, having a brain tumor is no small challenge (pun intended). My advantage was that I knew about my health issues before wanting to get pregnant, and thus, I could address them head-on. So, if you already have a diagnosis, take care of your health *now,* before you start trying to conceive. But maybe you had no idea something was wrong, and it was only because you were trying to conceive that you found out that your body was not functioning optimally. Whatever the case, please take heart—most women in our age group are in a similar boat.

It is an undeniable fact that the twenty-first century lifestyle I've mentioned in the preface has worn many of us down and weakened our bodies. Our food supply, our unhealthy lifestyle, all the toxins we are exposed to, and the improper use of the pill (the pill is often prescribed, not as a contraceptive, but as a way to get rid of menstrual cramps, headaches, breast tenderness, or mood swings, which are all signs of hormonal imbalances that should be properly addressed, not just masked) and other medications have taken a toll on many of us, including me. That's why we now see young women in their 30s showing signs of perimenopause (the natural transition into menopause), while, in previous generations, women underwent this transition in their 50s. Some of us age prematurely, and many of us have no idea what is really happening in our bodies. Until, that is, we decide to have children.

This is one of the biggest lessons I have learned on my own journey and through the interviews I've conducted: if you want to get pregnant later in life, you need to become the CEO of your body and of your health—ideally *before* you even try to conceive.

One startling example of a woman who took her destiny into her own hands and became the boss of her own health is functional nutritionist and hormone expert Alisa Vitti, who created the virtual hormone health center *FLOliving.com* and authored the bestselling book *WomanCode* (hands down, the best book I've read that easily breaks down the complexity of our female hormonal system and how it all relates to fertility). For the past seventeen years, Alisa has helped tens of thousands of women around the world resolve menstrual and fertility issues with her food-based protocol.

Her passion and drive for this topic was born out of necessity. When Alisa was in her early 20s, her doctor told her that she would have all kinds of issues in her life, including obesity and the propensity for diabetes, heart disease, and cancer. Oh, and also, she would never be able to naturally conceive. This was heartbreaking news for the young woman, especially since no doctor could tell her what was even wrong with her.

After seven long years, Alisa was finally diagnosed with a severe case of PCOS (the leading cause of infertility that affects up to10 percent of women in the United States) after *she* had done the research and suggested it to her doctors. At the time, Alisa was a student at John Hopkins University on her way to becoming an OB/GYN. She realized that traditional gynecology would not get her better, and so she turned to functional medicine (doctors and practitioners who address the whole person, not an isolated set of symptoms) and functional food (foods that have a potentially positive effect on health beyond basic nutrition).

Step by step, she got her health back. Alisa got her period on track, started sharing her knowledge, and built her practice in New York City before transforming it into the virtual FLOliving center (including the app MyFLO, the first functional medicine period tracker app that improves your period the more you use it) that has helped thousands of women from around the world resolve menstrual and fertility issues with her food-based protocol, a protocol she put to good use on herself as well. After getting married in 2012, Alisa and her husband were ready to start their family. At 37, she conceived her daughter naturally within only three months of trying.

"I wanted to take control of my body, and I wanted to do it naturally. That's why I am so passionate about sharing the science behind fertility and hormonal health," Alisa told me during our Skype chat between New York and DC. "Once women know they can improve their fertility and they get the information on what to do next, they can take action and prolong their fertility, instead of aging prematurely. Remember the times before the pill was invented, when women had their sixth, seventh, or eighth child at age 47 or 48? Women are meant to be optimally fertile for the maximum amount of time. We are designed to procreate the species and, as such, to be healthier longer and have a better immune system than our male counterparts."

"So why are so many couples today unable to conceive?" I asked.

"Even though we are designed to be fertile for a very long time, because of the chemicals in our environment and our stressful and often unhealthy lifestyle, we *have* to be proactive, we *have* to take action and not take it for granted that we can easily conceive like a woman several generations ago could. We have to protect and preserve our fertility!" (Please see the BODY Action Steps in chapter 14 for specific steps to take.)

Alisa overcame her serious disease, as did I and very many of the women I interviewed. So, if you, too, have had multiple miscarriages or an autoimmune disease or chronic illness, please know that you are not alone. And be assured that your diagnosis does not mean that you cannot, often dramatically, improve your health and, thus, your fertility (unless your condition is irreversible). As Alisa says, a woman is designed to be fertile for as long as possible, and your body has remarkable powers to heal itself.

Remember, the healthier you become, the higher your chances to conceive naturally or, if you should need assisted reproductive technology, to carry a healthy baby to term. So, if you have thoughts like, "My body is betraying me," or, "I cannot trust my body," or, "My body is turning on me," because you were diagnosed with a disease, then let me assure you: These thoughts come from our cultural beliefs and the idea that, if something bad happens to us, we must have done something wrong. And that's simply not true. You did not cause this. And luckily you can do a lot to help your body heal now.

You Are Not a Victim of Your Genes

"But what about my genes?" you may ask. Do you come from a family whose health record is less than stellar? If you do, I get it. My brother was diagnosed with Cushing disease when he was 17. His adrenal glands and two tumors in his brain needed to be surgically removed in subsequent years. My father died of pancreatic cancer. My mother had eight miscarriages and developed heart disease, breast cancer, *and* stomach cancer in her 70s and 80s. I've not inherited a spick-and-span genetic record either.

But, today, we know that the genes passed down to us from our family do not determine our future in the way we previously believed. In school, most of us learned the science of genetics. We were told that our genes determine the rest of our lives in regards to physical and emotional behavioral characteristics and health. But this is not true, as the newer study of epigenetics proves.

The science of epigenetics looks at how the environment and our lifestyle influences if and when our genes get turned on or off. Harvard- and MIT-educated MD Sara Gottfried, who happens to also be the *New York Times* bestselling author of *Younger*, makes this point: "We've learned through the study of epigenetics that you are not stuck with the genes you inherited. You can actually change the way your genes talk to the rest of your body. If you look at your risk of getting a disease, also degenerative diseases like cancer or heart disease, 10 percent is due to your genetics and 90 percent is due to your environment. What's key here is how much control you have with your small daily lifestyle choices to affect that 90 percent."

We Are Responsible *to* Our Health Challenges

We do not intentionally cause our illnesses, and there is no reason to blame ourselves for having developed these issues. I mean, really, who would deliberately want to cause an illness or create fertility challenges? So, if you already have experienced problems around your fertility, do not blame yourself for any issues. And please, don't blame yourself for having waited too long or start any other negative self-talk in your head or heart.

In the same token, we also need to acknowledge that, even though we are not responsible *for* our illnesses, we are responsible *to* our illnesses and to our fertility challenge. If illness or infertility shows up, we cannot just say, "Oh, my body is broken; I'll go to the doctor to fix it," as if we could detach ourselves from the vessel we are living in (an attitude which may be one of the reasons why the success rate of IVF is so low). Our bodies will nurture and grow a tiny egg into a full-fledged human being, so now is the time to truly "embody" the miracle we women are—not to intellectually separate from our bodies, the place our child will reside.

Our bodies are the manifestation of our beliefs, emotions, choices, and lifestyle. Our bodies usually don't get out of whack and fall into disease without us—often, unwittingly, we contribute to our own downfall. If we want to live an empowered life, we women need to take responsibility for our health, instead of handing responsibility over to our doctor or other health care provider. Even if you choose IVF down the road or are already undergoing treatment, you should take steps to improve your health. It will make you a better vessel for your child's development in utero and a healthier, more resilient mom. I strongly believe the idea that "my disease is out of my control" is the actual illness we need to treat.

Fall in Love with Your Body—It Won't Let You Down

There is also a chance that your physical fertility challenge may turn into an epiphany. "Disease," as I hear leading experts in female health say, "is the way our bodies can communicate with us." Some suggest that what happens with our bodies helps us to come into direct communication with our soul, our inner guide, our divine spark, if you will. Illness can very well be our bodies' way of getting our undivided attention so we can heal and become healthy again. Your body is incredibly resilient and won't let you down once you start believing in its innate strength.

Personally, I went beyond a cause-and-effect type of thinking and learned to relate to my cysts and fibroid in a new way. I bought Dr. Christian Northrup's book *Women's Bodies Women's Wisdom* and read up on the underlying emotional energy patterns that can contribute to a fibroid forming. When I read about fibroid tumors representing creativity that was never birthed, including "fantasy" images of ourselves that have never seen the light of day—and the idea that fibroids are often associated with conflicts about creativity, reproduction, and relationships—my curiosity was piqued. I contemplated Dr. Northrup's suggestions and found different ways to release my creativity.

I started to see my fibroid and cysts not as an enemy that needed to be conquered, but as aspects of my own inner guidance that were trying to direct my attention toward changes in my life that would actually enhance my health. I asked myself, "What is my body telling me?" and I followed up with an even better question: "What does my body need to become healthy and strong again?" Turns out, I did not need surgery or medication. For me, it was finding more creative outlets and starting a new career that had me travel and be giddily excited—*that* was what my body needed to heal and find balance again.

And, indeed, with time, the cysts and the fibroid went away by themselves. Even the MRI that I scheduled one year after the birth of my son revealed that there was no trace left of the brain tumor I was diagnosed with sixteen years earlier. In fact, the technician who did my scan commented that I have "a really beautiful brain." *Well, thank you.* It seems that the older I got, the healthier I became, just like Alisa and so many other women in this book.

Regardless of where you are in your journey to motherhood—contemplating getting pregnant in a few years or already in the thick of things—you need to look at your body as a friend who wants your help. When we all start to relate to our fertility in terms of our health (i.e., the healthier we are, the more fertile we are), instead of looking at it through the prism of age, we can then approach motherhood from a much more empowered and truthful standpoint because we can do something to improve our wellbeing. By making our bodies fertile soil, we can accomplish the following:

- Improve the quality of our eggs (and sperm, if your partner tunes up his health as well) and give our future children a better chance of being healthy. Excellent physical, emotional, and mental health of the parents means a better start for our babies, and it may even decrease the risk of chromosomal abnormalities.
- Boost our chance of having a healthy, strong, and essentially uneventful pregnancy that we can actually enjoy and cherish, rather than spending our time in fear that something could go wrong, even if we've experienced miscarriage(s) before (many of the women in this book, including myself, have).

- Set the stage for carrying the baby to full term and having a healthy delivery, regardless of our age. I naturally delivered at age 44, and it was the single-most empowering experience I've ever had. (Birth is one of life's events whose profound impact becomes clearer after some time has passed.)
- Are better able to bounce back from delivery and have more energy and vitality for raising our children. Being three years into living with a little one who calls me Mommy, I realize what a marathon motherhood truly is. And I strongly believe that we older moms owe it to our kids to be as vital and "long-lasting" as we can. (If you, too, are interested in getting "younger with age," check out my articles on this topic at *BettinaGordon.com*.)

Your health is paramount to conceiving, carrying to full-term, and raising your child. (Again, please read the BODY Action steps in chapter 14.)

Preparation Is Key, Especially at Our Age

First off, let me ask you a question: how long did it take you—or women you know—to plan your wedding? On average, how many hours per week did you spend flipping through magazines, researching venues, and checking on vendors? According to Wedding Paper Divas' survey, 47 percent of couples spend up to nine hours a week designing their wedding, and 40 percent spend up to fifteen hours a week—and the majority of couples have between thirteen to eighteen months between their yes and their I do. That's a whole lot of time spent getting ready for the big day.

So, what if I tell you that every single fertility expert I've spoken to said this: you and your partner should take a minimum of at least three, but ideally six to nine, months to prepare your body (and mind) for the other big day, the day you will conceive your child. Yes, like a vegetable garden that needs to be tended to and prepared before the seeds are even put in the soil, your body also needs to be prepared for the seed of your child. What are you thinking now? "Cool, I got this!" or, "Are you crazy? That much time to prepare our bodies before we even try to conceive?"

Preparation for conception is vital. If you are worried about your age and the passing of time, I recommend that you a) read the MIND pillar again and b) consider investing in a program with the right natural fertility specialist so that you can see faster results than if you go it alone. I also suggest this route for financial reasons: according to Advanced Fertility Center of Chicago, the average cost of IVF in the United States is currently about eleven- to twelve-thousand dollars, often significantly higher at prestigious centers. If you can prepare your body for the seed of your child to sprout at a fraction of that cost, I'd call that money well spent.

And even if you do have to go the IVF route after all, your egg quality will have improved and your healthy and strong body will be much better equipped to nurture and nourish your baby. You may need fewer rounds of IVF than you would have otherwise. Joining a program can make a critical difference for you. You find the natural fertility experts I personally trust and would go to for advice in this book and on my website *BettinaGordon.com*. Check out the interviews I've conducted so far with these experts, as this will give you a better understanding of who they are and how they interact with their patients—and if you find them to be a good fit for your personality as well.

If finances should prohibit you from participating in a program or working personally with a natural fertility expert, don't worry. By picking up this book, you are already way ahead of the curve and have gained a perspective other than what's out there in the mainstream media. In the MIND, BODY and SPIRIT Action Step chapters, you will get advice and recommendations that will considerably help to improve your chances to naturally conceive.

If you can, though, please don't try to do it all on your own. Assemble a support team—your sister, brother, mom, girlfriends, aunts, members in an online community, etc.—people who will encourage you and cheer you on. Join our community. Human love and connection is what makes us thrive and keeps us on target.

Assemble a Cheerleading Squad to Support You on Your Journey

Dr. Andrew Weil, integrative medicine practitioner and, for many, America's best holistic health guru, once said, "The primary bad powers of Western medicine is the ability of doctors to negatively influence the way a patient feels about her health." I can't even count how many times I've heard moms who are 40+ say how they were disrespected (Alicia: "'You should not have waited so long!' he scolded me in a snarky voice, as if I could have pulled my partner out of thin air!") or made to feel scared (Tricia: "'At your age, your risk of stillbirth skyrockets,' my doctor said, even though there was nothing in my pregnancy or my health chart that would suggest that.") or were treated in an aloof manner, like a number, without empathy or joy, let alone compassion and understanding.

Please hear me loud and clear on this one: You have knowledge of your body, and your doctor or nurse has a body of knowledge. If you merge these two, you can experience true health care and will have support and love (the most important ingredients next to having professionals with expertise on your team) on your journey to 40+ motherhood.

What we women on our fertility journey really need is this: we want to be heard, understood, and validated.

Why am I so strongly encouraging you to get your team together? We mature, "high-risk pregnancy" women are in a vulnerable place because we are constantly bombarded with negative headlines and statistics. We need to be proactive in order not to have our bodies fall victim to the "nocebo effect."

The medical establishment has been proving that the mind can heal the body for over fifty years with the so-called "placebo effect." We know from clinical trials that, when people are given a sugar pill or a saline injection or even a fake surgery, 18 to 80 percent of them get better. There are changes in the body that can be physiologically measured in the people who receive the placebo—bronchi dilate, warts disappear, colons become less inflamed. In Rogaine studies, bald guys on a sugar pill actually grew hair.

The other side of the coin, the evil twin to the placebo effect, if you will, is the nocebo effect. People participating in clinical studies are also informed of the harmful side effects they will experience when taking the drug—even if they only get the sugar pill. Science has found that just the thought that people might be at risk for these side effects actually makes them *get* these side effects. Even more startling, medical literature contains multiple test studies in which people who were told they were going to die within a certain amount of time because of, for example, cancer, died almost exactly to the date. My own father died pretty much at the six-month mark he was given by his doctors. However, here's the really bad part, which was thankfully not true for my father: there are a number of cases in which the autopsy reveals that the patients who died with a cancer diagnosis did not have cancer at all. How crazy and truly sad is that?

Dr. Lissa Rankin is a medical professional who has written about the power of mind-body unity. In her bestselling book *Mind over Medicine—Scientific Proof That You Can Heal Yourself*, Rankin, a former OB/GYN physician and the founder of the Whole Health Medicine Institute, writes about the in-depth studies conducted surrounding the placebo effect: "The researchers believe that some combination of the positive belief of the patients that they are going to get well and the nurturing care of somebody in a white coat saying, 'I believe this is going to help you,' is actually causing the healing." It is the combination of positive belief and the nurturing care of a health care provider that leads to changes in the brain that are translated into the physiology of the body through a whole cascade of hormonal changes.

I've often heard the women featured in this book say that they became pregnant only after they found their champion. Claudia Chan turned to Aimee Raupp for physical and emotional support. Margeaux ditched her cold and aloof infertility specialist—"He did not treat me as a person, but rather a case"—for another infertility specialist who was warm and funny and gave her hope that the new round of IVF could work. However, he never actually saw Margeaux again, as she was naturally pregnant before her next appointment. Denise worked with Alisa Vitti, Leah with Russell Davis, and Pippa with Andrew Loosely. I, myself, partnered at first with my doctor in Vienna and then with the midwives at the

George Washington University Hospital in DC, whose coveted program I joined as soon as I found out I was pregnant. The midwives never, not even once, brought my age up as a concern until the very end of my pregnancy, when I went past my due date.

When you assemble your cheerleaders, from your girlfriends to your medical team, consider also joining a group of other women wanting to get pregnant. If you do, you are more likely to conceive than if you are alone on your journey. And once you are pregnant, please know that a study published in the *Journal of the American Geriatrics Society* in November 2016 found that women who had a baby after the age of 35 were mentally sharper in old age—which means you *will* remember the location of your keys when it's time to drive to church for your grandchild's wedding.

Now that's news I can wholeheartedly get behind.

CHAPTER 9

Larissa

Sometimes heart connections are established in lightning speed and over a great distance. This is how I felt about Larissa, a New York City born and raised woman of Polish and Irish parents, who recently moved to Warsaw, Poland's capitol city. When I looked for forty women over 40 to interview for this book, I did not advertise the project on the internet or use my social media channels to promote it. It was not necessary, as the worldwide web brought them to me in amazing ways anyway. This time, the connection came through Kris Carr's Sexy Crazy B-School community[1], which Larissa and I belonged a year ago. Larissa found me through something I posted in this group, and a week later, we met for a heart-to-heart Skype chat.

By then, Larissa was one and a half years into her experience of motherhood, and she happily bounced her blond and blue-eyed son, Peter, on her knees. He was impressively chill throughout our one-hour talk. If I hadn't known that Larissa was 40 when she gave birth, I would have pegged her for a decade younger. With her black hair swept up in a ponytail, a slender frame, and an infectious smile, this mother defied anybody's stereotype about later motherhood. Like me, she was hesitant about becoming a mom—scars from her neglectful childhood

---

1   If you are not familiar with Kris Carr, please check her out. This woman is a beacon of light in the health and wellness industry: *KrisCarr.com*.

ran deep, and she wasn't sure she would be a good parent. But now, Larissa is a wonderful example of a woman who, in spite of her fear, decided to have a child anyway.

Larissa: Through most of my 30s, I was in a relationship with a man who was not right for me. I felt it in my heart, I knew it in my brain, but I could not get out of the relationship. I mean, I could, but I couldn't, if you know what I mean. I did think about children from time to time, but I was deeply afraid of making that commitment in general, let alone with the wrong partner. Eventually, I was able to break free from this toxic relationship, and as life would have it, within a year or so I met a wonderful man. Jan and I got married when I was 38, and I was very honest with him. I told him right away that, on the one hand, I would like to start a family, but on the other, I was afraid. He told me, "Of course, you are afraid; that's normal." He did not understand at first where I was coming from.

You see, I did not have the usual jitters that may come with big life choices like getting married or becoming pregnant. I was truly and deeply scared that my own upbringing might have messed me up too much to be a good mother to another human being. I had a chip on my shoulder. Whenever a woman told me she was pregnant, I would think to myself, "Really? You decided to bring a tiny human being into the world for whose safety, well-being, and happiness you are now completely responsible for over the next eighteen years?" I was sarcastic and overawed at the same time, but I knew that stemmed from not having had a very good experience myself as a child.

Bettina: What happened when you were young?

My family background was quite troubled, and I grew up with people who were fundamentally unhappy. My mom had a lot of mental illness and addiction problems—in many ways, I was not well looked after. It was imprinted into my young mind that it was difficult to care for a child. And it was certainly difficult for me as a child to deal with my parents' issues.

As an adult, I sought out things that helped me feel better about myself and that would build my confidence. For example, I joined Al-Anon, an organization that helps families and friends of alcoholics. I also went to therapy and took a course in alcohol counseling here in Poland that helped me better understand this addiction. For years, I'd been focused on personal development, and I'd been reading many wonderful books on the subject. I took a very active part in my betterment, choosing to do it for me, but also for the child I one day might bring into the world. When Jan and I married, I was already living in an empowered and much healthier way, both mentally and emotionally, but I still had not found the full confidence to say, "I can do this; I can be a good mom."

Looking at you today, with your boy in your lap, I would not have guessed that you had such trepidations. Did you just take a leap of faith, or did you approach pregnancy more methodically?

Well, I was still afraid I'd potentially mess my kid up, but I figured I'd start preparing to have one anyway *(laughs)*. I went to see a couple of doctors and had them check out my health, including my hormone status and thyroid levels, things like that. I started doing research online and found Alisa Vitti, who wrote the book *WomanCode*. She talks a lot about hormonal health and how we can naturally regulate our hormones by eating the right foods. There is quite a bit of information available on how to use nutrition to enhance fertility, but hardly anybody explains *why*.

Alisa, however, not only tells you that you need to support your liver and keep your blood sugar stable, but she explains why this needs to happen. So that really interested me, and I started to follow her recommendations—for example, I cut out caffeine. I was interested in Alisa's online courses, but when you live in Poland, you cannot afford many of the awesome resources available in the United States. The income disparity is just too significant.

But I found a Polish woman here who is a specialist in Chinese medicine, and she sat down with me for four hours and asked me the most amazingly detailed questions about every aspect of my life. And based on this, she produced a plan for me which was similar to Alisa's suggestions, but much more in depth. In general, I boosted my vegetable intake and avoided dairy products, caffeine, and sugar, and I also checked to see if I had a wheat sensitivity, something I had already suspected, as I felt tired whenever I ate wheat. I would totally feel bloated, which is ironic—wheat inhibits you from getting pregnant, but it makes you *look* pregnant *(laughs)*.

The same happens to me. I eat wheat, and my belly swells up like I am four months pregnant. I kid you not. I've actually been asked a couple of times if I *was* pregnant . . . darn wheat *(tries to laugh)*.

I so hear you. When I was in my 20s and early 30s, the same thing happened to me. But in order to get pregnant, I had to cut wheat out of my diet. So, I ate really clean for about seven months before we actively tried to conceive. When I tell this to people, I sometimes hear, "Oh, I could never give up my coffee or my wine or whatever. It would be too hard for me." It may feel scary at first, but once you get over that hump, it's not. It wasn't that difficult for me because I did not focus on what I was temporarily giving up, but on what I would gain in the long run. I guess there was a part of me that knew that I should prepare my body and make it as healthy as possible to have a healthy child.

Also, as difficult as my upbringing was, one of the good things my mom passed down to me was the habit of healthy eating. Mom was a doctor, and she taught me the value of nutrition. Oh, and I forgot to mention, I also went back into therapy during this time. I was seeing my therapist once a week, and it was really helpful to once again address my fears around motherhood and to work through them. You could say I made room for my child to come into my life by clearing psychic space and preparing my body.

Jan did not watch his diet the same way I did, but whenever we ate at home, which was the majority of the time, he would eat what I had prepared according to my diet. So, by extension, he was also very healthy. Then, a funny thing happened. I had unprotected sex with Jan twice in one weekend—it was the only time I had done so. And that's when I conceived. First, I thought, boy, that's what happens when you have unprotected sex. But if you look around, that's obviously not true. There are many couples struggling to conceive, and I cannot help but wonder if all the preparation I did, both physically as well as mentally, made the difference.

So, did you just gradually come to the moment of, "Let's go!" or was there a defining moment when you realized the time had come?

I'm glad you bring that up because there were actually two defining moments. The first one was a physical experience, and it was really strange. The month before I became pregnant, I had a very painful period—I mean, extraordinarily painful, which it never is. I was at work, and I suddenly started feeling nauseous and dizzy, and I had to throw up. My coworkers called an ambulance, and it took me straight to the hospital because the pain was so intense. At first, I thought it was a miscarriage, but it wasn't. But what was it? I have a good relationship with my body, and I believe my body speaks to me. So, I tuned into it and the message seemed to be, "Hello, wake up; I am here." My womb and this part of my body wanted to get my attention, and I guess it needed to be that loud for me to really hear it.

A couple of weeks later, I was listening to women's health pioneer Dr. Christiane Northrup on her Hay House radio show. A female listener called in, and she was talking about how desperate she was to get pregnant—and could Dr. Northrup or somebody, really anybody, help her? She was so sad, and I felt so sad for her, but it was also one of those moments that makes you think about yourself. It really kind of jolted me. There she was, truly sad and desperate, and it made me think, don't waste your chances, don't get yourself in a situation like hers. It was a clear sign to me not to miss my opportunity to have a family, not to let fear stand between me and my child any longer. In hindsight, it was then that the pull toward pregnancy became much stronger than my fear. I was ready.

Ready and pregnant in no time. How was the pregnancy? And, more important, how is being a mother?

I remember the pregnancy as being wonderful, even though the first trimester was tough. I was tired, threw up, and had some bleeding, so the doctor put me on bedrest for six or seven weeks, which is not unusual here in Poland. I wasn't lying in bed all day, but I was off from work and took it easy. He also made me take synthetic progesterone, which I was worried about since I know you can naturally boost progesterone through the food you eat. But maybe I needed a higher intensity, and so I took it, and all went well.

The second and third trimester were fantastic, and I felt strong and beautiful. In the first trimester, I had eaten whatever I craved, mainly bread and such, but I consumed foods that were good for the baby's development, things like Brazilian nuts and sweet potatoes, for the rest of the pregnancy. I wish there would be a great book about what to eat when you are pregnant. Peter was born healthy and strong two weeks after my 40th birthday.

As for motherhood now? It is so amusing, because all the things that I was *not* worried about—fatigue, the effort of establishing a new business from home since I did not want to go back to my old job, or the sheer madness of finding the right nanny to help me with Peter—are the things I now grapple with. As for my previous fears? I am so busy, I don't even have the time to sit and contemplate the responsibilities of being a mom. Funny, huh? Every now and then I think, "Wow, look at the world around us. How do we bring up a happy child?" but I don't feel isolated—I have support. I still go to therapy, and I still have friends I have very open conversations with, like we are doing right now. I found that a lot of things come naturally to me as a mother and that I am able to figure things out. I do my best, and I increasingly feel that that is good enough for my Peter, if you know what I mean.

Are you two thinking about having a second child?

Yes, I started to ramp up my diet already and was planning to try to conceive soon, but my dad was recently diagnosed with cancer, and it does not look good. It doesn't seem to be a good time for me to be pregnant with all that is going on in my family. Even though I, in general, have no issues with my age—in fact,

Larissa

I find motherhood in my 40s pretty perfectly timed—for a short time, I was panicking that I am now over 40 and need to hurry. Can I really see my father through this and wait until next year to get pregnant? So, it's nice to talk to you and remember that I don't need to panic, that there is so much we can do to enhance and prolong fertility. I just need to look after myself the same way I did before and trust it will happen again. Also, by then, maybe I will be a little less tired *(laughs)*.

CHAPTER 10

Darviny and Bernadette

One thread that continued through many of my interviews was especially fascinating to me: women who, in their younger years, were diagnosed with a physical disorder like PCOS or who did not get pregnant despite having "young and wild" unprotected sex with their first husbands became more fertile with age and fell pregnant at 43, 44, 45, or even 46. (Their exes, by the way, also frequently went on to become fathers.) Since I do believe that we women know our bodies the best, I was more than happy to connect with Darviny and Dr. Bernadette, as both women hold a unique and powerful perspective on their pregnancies.

Darviny is a former restaurateur, fashion designer, boutique owner, yogi, and artist who now reinvents herself on the internet as a lifestyle connoisseur. Just Google her name, and you will find multiple projects that this blonde-haired extrovert has launched. When I Skyped with Darviny from her home in the Florida Keys, she was dressed in a colorful outfit with wild patterns and a pink headband wrapped around her long mane.

Born to French parents, Darviny has a deep love for all things European, so we both hit it off right away. I also liked Darviny's straightforward attitude and that at her age (she was 53 at the time or our talk, 45 when she became a mother), she does not seem to care what others think. She owns her feminine power and raises her daughter accordingly. Somehow, it was not a surprise to hear that this woman had not planned on having kids with her second husband—her life had been very full and rich to begin with.

Darviny: Some women make having babies a priority, but I always felt that, if it happens, it happens, and if it doesn't, that's fine too. I did not need to have children to be complete. When Tom and I married, we figured we'd live an "adult life," with lots of international travel, work, and play. We had talked about children, but since I had never conceived in all the years of unprotected sex with my first husband, I figured I could not naturally get pregnant. And I was vehemently against injecting my body with hormones and drugs. The doctors really push fertility treatments and C-sections on us women down here. It's really bad. I have friends who were 30 and 31 years old and still newlyweds when their doctor pushed them into IVF because they were young and had not gotten pregnant within one year. In Miami, it seems like it does not matter if you are young or old, the doctors shove their treatments on you, regardless. Anyway, she drank the Kool-Aid and ended up with triplets! I was not up for that, and Tom was fine with not having kids as well.

Bettina: And yet, at age 45 you birthed your healthy daughter, Alexandra, whose smiling face I've seen in the photos you post. You both look genuinely happy.

And we are! The pregnancy was a *huge* surprise to me and Tom, and yet, in hindsight, I see how I inadvertently may have broken through the mental barriers that kept me from previously conceiving. During the first summer that Tom and I were newly married, I was driving up the highway from the Keys to my art studio in Miami. I was listening to a radio show that talked about how, when you plant a seed, you don't see the seed grow, but it is still doing its thing under the dirt in the ground. And eventually it becomes something that flourishes and breaks through the soil for all to observe. The radio host connected this conversation to a woman's body and a pregnancy, how the fertilized egg starts growing without the woman even knowing it.

I was listening to this and imagining how that must happen and how you don't know that new life is growing inside of you. And I was going on this whole tangent of listening—but I mean really, really listening—to this show. I remember thinking, "Wow, nature is just amazing." You know how we can go into a trance when we are driving a route that we know like the back of our hand? I became completely absorbed, and I thought about nature and how there is a baby forming and that there is a heartbeat and little fingers and organs being created, and the woman may not even know until she's eight, nine, ten weeks along. What a miracle!

So, I went off on twenty minutes of "wowness" of listening to the show, and I now believe that this experience opened me up subconsciously, clearing a mental block that I had had. I think that our minds are really powerful, without us actually realizing how powerful they truly are. I was not calling a pregnancy in, but I was off on a total daydream, in amazement of the female body, of my body. I kept thinking, "Aren't our bodies amazing? This body is made for me and look what can happen. Imagine if that would happen to me; imagine I wouldn't even know!" These were the thoughts that I had, and I was in complete awe. I strongly believe this experience was the priming for things to come.

According to studies, 91 percent of our thoughts are actually in the subconscious. You think that this experience cleared up a subconscious mental block around pregnancy that you were not consciously aware you had?

Yes, that's right. I did not want to have children because I did not want to do fertility treatments. The underlying thought was that I could not get pregnant anyway. I did not believe my body could do it. Then I listened to the radio show that was all about the miraculous female body, and I went away from this experience in awe about the things my body could do. And I really think that, if women who are trying to become pregnant could unblock their subconscious and open up to the universe, it would allow the energy for pregnancy to come in. But that's a whole other story.

Shortly after the show, I flew to France, where I have a house, for the summer. Tom needed to work, so he stayed stateside, and I went to work wholeheartedly on my art in my studio there. I was creating a beautiful collection on large sheets of paper, the same as Picasso had used, and I was showing and selling my art in France. I was loving this summer, and I was fully engaged and present in my life. I lived in the moment and loved what I was doing. I was really alive, if you will. We often think of fertility as being a physical attribute, but as women, we are fertile in so many ways, and being creative opened up my second chakra, the chakra that is located in the lower belly and represents the reproduction zone. It was wide open, not because I was having sex, but because I was creating and loving what I did. I created some fertile soil that summer, let me tell you *(laughs)*, and it was one of my best collections ever!

Well, the best was actually yet to come. Tom was scheduled to visit for one week, and coincidentally, I had a friend come to visit with her four children at the exact same time. We had dinner parties and kids and visitors and an all-in-all crazy week. Tom and I only had sex once during his visit. Once. And I did not think anything of it until I returned to America a month and a half or so later. I had gained a little weight and so had Tom. We both went on a super healthy diet, and he lost weight, but I did not. I thought, huh? That was the first time I realized that I could be pregnant.

Did you fall off the toilet seat when you saw the blue lines on your test?

Absolutely. In fact, I even snuck out of the house that morning and rushed to my OB/GYN, who is also a good friend, to confirm the result with a blood test. When I told Tom, he was dumbfounded. First, he said, "Very funny." Then he asked me if I had had an affair in France, which was even funnier. I mean, who gets pregnant at 44 ½ with one time? By then I was nine or ten weeks along already . . . and I had not known, just like on the radio show!

My pregnancy was a most wonderful experience. I was in pretty good shape before I got pregnant, as I am a passionate cook and love to prepare healthy, fresh meals, and I believe my health helped me get pregnant so easily. Once I was pregnant, however, I lost my shape *(laughs)*, as I gained sixty pounds. I still ate healthy, just much more than usual, and I also took long walks on the beach and put my feet up whenever I wanted. I celebrated my pregnancy, and it was a most wonderful experience that I never would have wanted to miss![2]

Next, I'd like to introduce you to Bernadette.

When my friend, Michaela, offered to put me in touch with Dr. Bernadette Stringer, I immediately jumped at the opportunity. Bernadette is one person I was "über eager" to talk to because she embodies a story literally every single one of us has heard before: a woman who cannot get pregnant adopts, and voila, shortly thereafter, she becomes pregnant herself.

It took a few weeks to track this busy lady down, but when we spoke, it was like I'd found a woman I would like to go on an adventure with, riding camels through the Sahara or gliding in hot air balloons over Turkey. Bernadette, a pediatrician who runs a very well-regarded hospice for children in Austria's "Sound of Music" city, Salzburg, is fun, thoughtful, and full of life. She has a no-nonsense, thoughtful demeanor, and I was glad I had the chance to ask her how her story unfolded and why she thought she got naturally pregnant at 43, three years after she was told she had a 0.1 percent chance of ever conceiving.

Bernadette: Having children was always part of my life's plan. I love them and think children are great fun. I even chose to become a pediatrician and dedicate my career to research and to running the oncology department of large hospitals. I did want to have a family, just not right away. I was in my mid-30s when I met my now husband, who is ten years older and who already had two children with his first wife. He was originally done with having children. Thankfully, he changed his mind. He thinks I would have been deeply unhappy if I would not have had the chance to experience motherhood and have my own family. There is truth to that.

---

2   Read more about how Darviny raises her daughter, Alex, as a global citizen in "*SISTERHOOD*," which you'll find at *BettinaGordon.com*.

Bettina: So, you tried to get pregnant but could not?

Exactly. I reached out to a friend of mine who is an OB/GYN and sought his advice. I was pretty adamant that I did not want to go overboard with multiple rounds of IVF and such, but I wanted to know my options. I was diagnosed with primary (also referred to as premature) ovarian failure. We did two rounds of IVF, and even with the high dosage of hormones required for IVF, no useful eggs ripened. I also did one special therapy with an ultra-high hormone dosage, and nothing happened.

It became clear that all the reproductive medicine in the world could not help me. The doctors told me that maybe I would have had a good chance of conceiving in my early 20s, but even back then, I might have had difficulties. I had no idea about any of this—I had always menstruated regularly and normally. I was even able to feel when I ovulated—the eggs being released were simply not good enough to sustain a pregnancy. Now, at age 40, I was told that my chances of getting pregnant spontaneously, meaning naturally, was 0.1 percent and that each month that passed, these chances got even lower.

Were you devastated by the news?

I was deeply saddened that I would not experience a pregnancy. I was grappling with the fact that everything in my life had gone very well, but that this one topic, my own family, was not within my reach. I was also wondering if it was okay and fair to a child to become a mother at 40. Would it still be good and authentic to be in your mid-50s when your child enters puberty? Was it even acceptable to have a child so late? I wrestled with these thoughts. And I wrestled with my conscience.

As another option to conceive, we looked at egg donations, something that I did not initially consider. I now very much understand how a woman, how a couple, could get sucked onto this path so easily, especially when wanting a baby becomes the dominant thought in their lives. But I had to put the brakes on, as this option was simply too spooky to me. How could I explain to my child that somewhere there was a woman who got paid money to donate her eggs to create my child with my husband's sperm, that I had been the surrogate mother to my own child during pregnancy? This was not the right way for me. However, I also want to say very clearly that I do truly understand if a woman goes that route and that I do not judge her choice. It was just too weird for us.

What saved my sanity was the fact that we were simultaneously looking into adoption, an option that I had thought about since my teenage years. I had never felt like I needed a biological child or to pass on my "awesome" genes. I wanted a child but whether it was related through blood or not was not a concern for me. My husband and I picked South Africa and started to work with a reputable agency, as it was immensely important to us that the children were truly given up for adoption and not kidnapped or paid for. In February 2007, when I was 41, we welcomed our five-month-old boy from Johannesburg. And I joined the ranks of the older moms *(laughs)*.

So, now we have entered the classic story of a woman who is not able to get pregnant, but soon after she adopts, that's exactly what happened. Is this your tale?

You know, I had friends say to me, "You'll see; now that you are relaxed, it'll happen." And even my husband said, "When you are relaxed, we could do another round of IVF if you'd like." I heard it all, but truthfully, I was done. I was very happy with our son, and I had accepted that no biological child would be joining us. My struggle to conceive now made sense to me—this is how I had to find my son. And I was fine. We did start a second adoption process, but the door to natural pregnancy was closed.

When our son joined our family, I stayed home for a year. Gradually, I went back to work. Then we went on a family vacation in Greece, and I remember that I was utterly tired and exhausted. I was back to working seventy to eighty hours a week, but I now also had a husband, a son, a garden, etc. Of course I was tired! I was actually a bit afraid I had leukemia or something.

When we came home, my husband noticed that I bought ten glasses of pickled mushrooms, something that I had never done before, and devoured them with salt and lemon. He encouraged me to take a pregnancy test, which I did. I secretly did the test in our bathroom and then forgot about it for hours because I was hosting a dinner party. When I finally saw it, I could not believe it—almost three years after I was told I had a 0.1 percent chance of conceiving and that those chances were diminishing with every month, I was, indeed, pregnant.

I don't think my pregnancy was a result of being more relaxed, because the pressure of getting pregnant to have a child was long gone. It had been gone for almost two years. If anything, I was under even more pressure and stress professionally, because I had returned to my job and worked as much as before, in addition to having and caring for my little boy. I don't have any definitive proof, but I don't think my pregnancy happened because I was less stressed. I believe that motherhood itself affected my hormones. I could see how me stepping fully into my new role as a mother, embracing all the emotions, duties, and joys wholeheartedly, could very well have influenced my body.

The medical community acknowledges that a woman's body can become more fertile after she's birthed a child. But you are saying that simply having a child, your adopted son, may have had the same effect on your body?

Yes. What reproductive medicine failed to achieve—balancing my hormones and making my body produce quality eggs that could create life—motherhood and caring for my little son may have made possible. I don't know if it's true, but this is my theory, and it makes sense to me. I birthed my daughter one month before my 44th birthday, and she is perfectly healthy and a joy to be around.

I have thought about this experience of conceiving naturally quite a lot, and I think that doctors, and human beings in general, tend to look for reasons why something is happening. But maybe, in the end, it does not matter. It is what it is.

CHAPTER 11

Pippa and Denise

There are bad things that happen in everybody's life. And then there are the tragedies that can derail a person for many years to come. Pippa was a 29-year-old, happily married woman with the dream of starting her own family when her father took his own life. His suicide—he had suffered from a severe case of tinnitus, a loud ringing noise in his head that he could no longer cope with—left the whole family devastated and knocked his daughter firmly off course. "My father's suicide left me very vulnerable and insecure, like I did not have the strength to gain independence," Pippa told me during our Skype chat. "So, I became my mother's caretaker. Even though I live one-hundred miles away, I was seeing her all the time, taking care of her, and supporting her. For some people who experience a bereavement like this, a child can bring new hope and uplift them, but because this was a particularly difficult time for me, I felt I couldn't take the risk of making such a huge life change."

To add another dimension to an already difficult situation, Pippa suspected that, traced back to its roots, her father's suicide was connected to his own upbringing. "I believe that the reason why he could not cope with his illnesses was a lack of resilience that came from the poor parenting he received as a child. So, I felt that, as a mother, I needed to be in a place where I could offer really,

really good parenting to my child so that he would have the strength to survive all that life would throw at him."

Once she felt that her own mother was stable, Pippa went to work on herself. She signed up for personal therapy and even became a counselor herself. Today, at age 44, Pippa looks and speaks like the capable, mature, and confident mother she set out to be. After her father's death, it had taken her six years to come back to her original dream of starting a family and another seven years to, at 42, hold her newborn son in her arms.

Pippa: At age 35, we gave it a try, but nothing happened. My doctor told us not to worry and to just relax. We were both healthy and figured, hey, we can do it on our own. But, at 39, we were still trying. I knew all the literature said that I was getting old and that I would have problems conceiving. So, the pressure started to build, and for the first time, the thought, "Maybe it's not going to happen," set in.

Eventually, we had some tests done, and this was a really unpleasant experience. There was negativity surrounding my age and our counselor, who was a high-ranking expert in the field, had awful people skills. He treated me as if I were an anonymous object, showing an utter lack of compassion and sensitivity. This left me feeling frustrated and unvalued. He also had a very small selection of things to offer and simply pushed us toward IVF, which did not feel right to us. I did not want to force something that should happen naturally. The thought of creating a child in a test tube made me think, maybe we weren't meant to have children. IVF just did not sit well with me.

Bettina: Did you get any definite diagnosis?

They did not find anything wrong, so we were given this label of "unexplained infertility." But I questioned this diagnosis—just because pregnancy hasn't happened yet doesn't mean that a couple is infertile! It seemed like a really strange diagnosis to give. They could not show me that I was infertile, so I refused to take it on as truth. When I got close to 41, a friend sent me the link to a fertility online summit through which I heard Andrew Loosely speak for the first time.

After listening to a few of his talks, I became interested in working with him—I was so impressed by what he said. His people skills were really good and respectful; there was no judgment, no negativity, and his success rate was over 70 percent. Most of his clients were over 40, and I liked the Traditional Chinese medicine philosophy of a woman being fertile until menopause. He knew so much information that, in comparison, the people I had seen before, the ones who were supposed to be the experts, didn't seem to know anything.

What did Andrew suggest you do that the other doctors did not?

He looked at me from a holistic point of view and helped me strengthen my overall health to boost my fertility. Since my husband and I received a clean bill of health, I intuitively felt that maybe something was going wrong either at conception or implantation—a suspicion Andrew later confirmed when he looked at my detailed blood panel. In a nutshell, Andrew wanted to make sure I was strong enough for the whole process. That made a lot of sense to me, even though, honestly, after seven years of trying, I was so used to being disappointed month after month that I doubted it would actually work. Funny, huh?! I had strong doubts and a limited amount of money, only enough to work with Andrew for about six or seven months.

So, you doubted it would happen. How did you cope with the idea of maybe never becoming a mother?

It was kind of a despair and desolation but not as if I wouldn't be able to survive without a child. It was more like, "Oh, I have to find another thing in my life that will give me fulfillment and satisfaction in the way that a child would have." My husband and I were on the same page here: we needed to find other ways to feel fulfilled. Maybe we'd find a project together or find other ways of growing, of being creative, of finding joy. When I started my training to become a priest, I actually thought that it was my substitution for a baby *(laughs)*. The training made me feel that my life was really worthwhile. Priests give a lot, but they also get back a lot too, and there are many emotional highs. Training for priesthood gave me new challenges; it made me grow. And I always thought that there should be women priests, so this also motivated me and gave me satisfaction and fulfillment.

Do you think that having this new outlet to feel fulfilled and challenged may also have contributed to your fertility?

Sure. We also went on a lot of retreats to beautiful settings and amazing gardens, where the meals were all prepared for us and we were in silence, without the stress and hectic existence of daily life. I came back floating around, and everybody was noticing how peaceful I was. Also, there was something interesting that happened at church one day. There was a woman in her 60s, whom I told about my fertility troubles, and quite out of the blue, she said, "If you want to make it happen, it will happen!" That startled me. And I thought, maybe I need to be more proactive and grab my chance now, instead of just waiting for it to arrive. I had been concentrating on all the negative statistics about my age and the likelihood that I only had a 5 to 10 percent chance of conceiving, and her words were so refreshingly different!

So, I really dove into my work with Andrew over Skype. He taught me how to eat really well. He said I needed to sleep more and keep warm and reduce stress. He taught me things to avoid and things to seek out. He told me to keep my fertile areas warm. I was wearing thermal underwear quite a lot, and I no longer had cold feet and hands. I started to feel really, really good after only a couple of months, and I had more energy. My self-care was much, much better with him than before.

Sure, I needed a lot of discipline to follow through with all of his suggestions, like cutting out alcohol, coffee, sugar, and refined starches, but the changes I experienced were tremendously motivating. I added lots of green vegetables to my diet, and after having been a vegetarian for twenty years, I started to eat chicken and meat again, which Andrew encouraged me to do. I now eat liver and everything else and feel so much better than I previously did. All these changes, in combination with the herbs that Andrew personally prescribed for me, made a tremendous difference in my life.

I also benefited from my personal development work and my training for priesthood. I became really strong, very resilient, and emotionally secure, and I knew that, even if I'd never become a mom, I'd be sad, but I'd still be okay. I was on Andrew's program for six months and felt great, but I did not get pregnant. Then Andrew said, "One more month," and that's when it happened!

After seven years of trying, you were pregnant within seven months with Andrew?

Yes! I had a dream about having a baby about two weeks before I found out. I was elated. My husband nearly collapsed; he was so happy and amazed. Nothing has been the same after that. Especially when we saw the first scan and heard the heartbeat—it was so amazing. My pregnancy was great because I was super healthy, and I loved being pregnant. I continued this way of eating until now, two years after birthing my boy, because I feel so much better.

My husband and I were married for seventeen years when we became parents, and I think it's much easier for us to cope, as we know each other so well. How people who only know each other for a year or two do it, I don't know, because it's so demanding. Our child brought us closer together, and we are rather relaxed parents, rarely stressed or anxious. I think that, because we waited so long, we really appreciate and cherish our time together as a family. If I would advise another woman dealing with a similar situation, I would tell her to look into Traditional Chinese medicine because that takes the pressure off of your age. I'd also encourage her to look beyond the normal medical system for better information and to find people who can really support and value her! Whatever treatment she chooses, it should enhance her life, not weaken it.

Meet Denise, whose family tree suggested an easy pregnancy.

Just like my own grandmother, Denise's grandmother delivered her youngest child when she was in her 40s. So, naturally, Denise, who lived in wellness-obsessed, sunny California and followed a pretty healthy lifestyle all throughout her adulthood, figured that the combination of good genes and good lifestyle would mean an easy pregnancy at age 41. When her husband suggested preliminary tests just to confirm that her reproductive organs were firing on all cylinders, Denise thought it unnecessary. But eventually she agreed and made an appointment with her gynecologist. It was just a formality, right? I especially love Denise's story, as it shows that there is always room for improvement and that even something so small as picking up a book at the local bookstore can change a life forever.

Denise: I didn't believe I needed to get tested because my grandmother had my uncle when she was 46, and so I figured my eggs were fine. My cycle and everything had always been totally normal my whole life. But when I made my appointment with my gynecologist, she told me that, judging from my age and the statistics, she already knew what my hormone levels were going to be. I couldn't believe she would say that, as I knew I was eating really well and assumed I would have perfect levels. When we got the test results back, I was shocked to hear that I had an FSH level of fifteen. This was not horrible, but it meant that my ovaries were barely producing good eggs and that I'd have a 5 to 8 percent chance of conceiving naturally.

This came out of nowhere for me—I didn't even know what an FSH level was. It was all very curt and very scientific and heavy. She gave me the name and number of the local IVF guy. I couldn't even get a word in. I was so bombarded with this news. I already felt like she didn't know what she was talking about. I had overcome things before, like horrible acne in my 30s, and I figured that out on my own. So, I did some research and called her back. I asked her if I might be able to change the levels. She said that FSH could not be changed, and I partially believed her. Here's this trained doctor telling me I'm done, that I waited too long—that I'm 41 and it's over. All I had at that time was my pop-culture knowledge, all these celebrities who had had children at my age or older. She told me they're all having twins, and there's a reason for that: they're having IVF.

At this point, I didn't know anything about my cycle. I knew there was the menstrual cycle and that I ovulated, but that was it. I did some simple research online and found this woman who has a fertility cookbook, which tells you all the things you can do, like eat really plain foods and lots of avocados. It wasn't very scientific, and I'm an insane Virgo—I need to know why everything is happening, and I need to know the facts in order to keep me motivated. And so, I disregarded it, and for about a year after my test, I was just going about my business. I live in an area of Southern California with great craft beers, so every weekend was full of beer for me. I was eating a lot of meat and a lot of cheese. Getting pregnant was on the backburner. I wasn't taking control over my diet in a real way.

Bettina: So, what changed? What put your firmly on your path to parenthood?

Around the end of August 2013, I was at a local bookstore and saw the purple cover of *WomanCode* by Alisa Vitti. For whatever reason, maybe because I was supposed to buy it, I grabbed it, and I started reading the fertility section. I decided to purchase the book right then and there. I burned through it and realized, "Okay, I now see what I have to do." I loved the testimonials. I knew they had to be true. So, I decided to follow the steps in the book. I got rid of the sugar, cheese, and gluten. Now I'm making amaranth pasta with no cheese. I got rid of all the wine and all the beer. By the time my birthday came around and I turned 42, I decided to do it exactly as written for ninety days, and I synced the food I ate with the four phases of my menstrual cycle, just as Alisa describes in the book.

I went back to the same gynecologist after those ninety days. I asked to get my levels checked again. She didn't want me to get my hopes up because, at that point, it was a year later, which I get. They have people come to their office who are hopeful, but they don't know what to do or how to change a result. I told her I was doing this diet specifically for my cycle. I told her I was eating in sync with my cycle and that I'd gotten rid of all the inflammatory foods and instead was eating fertility-boosting foods.

She didn't understand what I was talking about, but she took my blood again and called me two days later. She said, "You need to hear this. It's as if I'm looking at the results of a completely different person. Your FSH is 7.5. That's the normal level of a healthy 33-year-old. You're 42. This shouldn't have happened. What did you do exactly? And what's the name of the book?"

That's outstanding. Congratulations!

Thanks. But now I was arrogant. I called all my friends and told them my results. I told everyone with fertility issues to do this diet and that it works. With an FSH level of 7.5, I was thinking, "I've got this in the bag." Just to show you how sensitive our bodies are, let me tell you what happened next. I started having some bread and a beer a week. A few weeks later, when I was still not pregnant, I decided to get myself tested again. Even though I was still eating in sync with the phases of my cycle and I ate buckwheat, avocados, brazil nuts, tons of vegetables, making brown rice and turmeric, and putting cinnamon on everything . . . well, my FSH went up to 9.8.

Alisa says that women are hormonally very sensitive these days because of the pesticides in our food supply, our lifestyle that's taxing our endocrine system, and the fact that we are delaying motherhood. So, this new test result got me right back on track, and I started to rigorously stick to the diet again. I did it to have a baby, but also because I had realized that all the symptoms of PMS that I had previously experienced—my depression and rage before my period—had all gone away within three months of being on the *WomanCode* program. No more cramping and no more bloating.

It was like I was 16 again. I just had my period, and it was done, without any problem. I felt so good. People were asking me what I was doing. They thought I had gone vegan. Everyone was wondering why I looked so good. I was telling everyone to get this book, as I was living proof it worked! Who doesn't want to feel their best all of the time?

Interestingly, I also noticed how my voice changed while being on the protocol. I am a professional singer, and my singing became crystal clear. There was no blockage. I think it had to do with getting rid of all the inflammatory food. My tone was clean because my body was clean. I also got rid of all the cleaners I had at home and other endocrine disruptors, like my moisturizer. It was a moisturizer from this place in New York that I paid fifty dollars for, and I had such a hard time getting rid of it. I wanted to give it away, but I knew it was an endocrine disruptor, and I couldn't give it to someone, knowing what it could do. So, eventually, I tossed it after all.

How long did it take for you to conceive after following Alisa's protocol?

Only four months! And I am thrilled to report that my child is healthy as can be. Because I was 43 when I was pregnant, my doctor made me do all this genetic screening, and I heard all about the chances of having a Down syndrome child or a child with severe genetic defects. When we got the results back, they were expecting them to be horrible. When we crunched the numbers, this one woman, who was initially really negative, couldn't believe what she saw. She said that we did not even need an amnio with these results. She said, "A healthy 16-year-old would have the same results as you!" The genetic testing doesn't factor in once you've done the protocol. Now I'm this crazed woman telling everyone about it—eating for fertility and health really works!

CHAPTER 12

Elise

Elise and I were introduced through my father-in-law during a trip to Chicago, and we bonded over our joint passion for healthy food for our boys. So, while Elise, the vegetarian, and me, the omnivore, talked shop about organic lentil dishes, Brussels sprouts recipes, and the supermarket ALDI's latest organic products (if you don't know ALDI, check them out—more and more they have high-quality organic products for low prices), we naturally transitioned into talking about our families. At age 46, Elise came to motherhood even later than I did. Previously married for twenty years without ever falling pregnant, Elise was not even sure she could conceive a child—or wanted to, for that matter. But her motherly instincts awoke when she started dating Arnoux and observed him caring for two-year-old Lilly, who was—wait for it—his grandchild.

"We were both in love with Lilly and seeing him interact with her awoke in me the wish to start a family," Elise remembers. Quickly, the blonde, brown-eyed American and the statuesque, black South African became a committed couple. And for Elise, the idea of motherhood and having a baby—something she had not really considered before—slowly grew into a deep desire. Simultaneously, Arnoux, initially excited about marrying and having a baby with his new love, slowly cooled off on the idea of starting all over again. I found Elise's example especially interesting: how do you navigate the waters of starting a family when the partners bring decades of marriage (not to each other), kids, grandkids, and two very different cultures into the mix?

Elise: I was barely in my 20s when I got married to a man I would spend two decades with. It was not a bad relationship by any stretch of the imagination, but it also wasn't a strong relationship—there was no deep connection between the two of us. My ex-husband and I are still friends, yet when we were married, we had years where I would be more committed than he was and vice versa. He is a very analytical person, and I am emotional—I feel deeply. And I never felt that he and I were truly connected. That may explain why I never got pregnant in the twenty years we were together, despite the fact that we did not use contraception. At some point, I wondered if there was an issue with me, and I brought it up with my OB/GYN in passing, but she basically shrugged her shoulders and did not order any tests. Today, I know that she could have easily done some noninvasive exams, but back then, I was not aware of the options, and I dropped the topic.

So, I focused more on my career and made progress in my work. I set myself the goal to earn a PhD and happily plugged along. Funnily enough, though, career has never been my top priority, neither then, nor now. I think I focused on it because my marital relationship was not that strong. If things would have been better between us, we may have had a child or two and probably would have stayed married. But since our relationship was mostly out of sync, I can't help but wonder if the writing was on the wall. On an unconscious level, I may have known that he was not the right man to have a child with. I remember wondering to myself what kind of father he would be.

Bettina: How did you eventually meet the man with whom you wanted to have a child?

Arnoux and I met when he hired me as a social worker for the mental health clinic he worked for at that time. We were both married and would occasionally socialize. Over the years, we established a friendship, and when my husband and I finally split, I would go on dates from time to time and tell Arnoux about them afterwards, which is rather funny in hindsight. It was nice that we had a chance to establish a friendship and mutual connection before we became a couple.

At some point, I realized that Arnoux and his wife were living separate lives and that his sons were all grown up and had left the house. Eventually they divorced, and Arnoux moved into a townhouse by himself. And then there was this night, you know one of those nights when you had a little too much to drink and you think, "Oh, what the heck," and then you discover a whole new side to the other person, a side you had never known. I had not seen his passionate side, and I must say, I liked it. A lot *(laughs)*.

I was very intrigued, and we started spending quality time together. Arnoux grew up in South Africa, in a traditional Christian family. When he came to America, it was a natural extension of his culture to marry a South African lady and start a family in his late 20s. So, when he and I finally became a couple, Arnoux was already a grandfather, and he would take wonderful care of his granddaughter, Lilly, who was about two years old at the time.

I had a chance to observe him with this small child and saw how lovingly he interacted and how he adored the little girl. And I myself fell in love with Lilly as well. The three of us would do things together, and I kept asking to see her almost every weekend that we spent together. We would also have her sleep over, and I immensely enjoyed her company. She was such a wonderful little girl. Lilly brought the mothering instinct out in me, and I could not get enough of her. She also prepared me for motherhood, which I started to hope for. Something that didn't seem possible all of a sudden became an option.

How did Arnoux react? Was he easily willing to start all over again?

In the honeymoon phase of our relationship, he absolutely was. Even though he had two grown sons, he was like, "Sure, we can get married and have a baby," and I totally bought into it. I got excited, and for the first time in my life, I could actually see it happening; I could see becoming a mom and raising a child. The more enthusiastic I got, the longer it took me to realize that Arnoux's interest in starting a new family was waning. I did not see it at first, but when I eventually caught on, our relationship took some hard turns. I got nervous. Here I was, 40+ years old, hoping to become a mom and have a child with this man, and all of a sudden, I found myself in a relationship with him that I was not sure would survive.

At the same time, the idea of going through the rest of my life without having experienced being a mom became daunting and scary. What would life be worth if I didn't experience that? I got anxious and reached out to friends who assured me that, if motherhood was something I wanted to experience, I could do it, even without Arnoux. Not that it would be easy, but that there were options, and I felt encouraged to explore them. I started to think about adoption and looked at adopting from another country or through the foster care system. And then I made an appointment at one of Chicago's leading fertility clinics.

How old were you at that time, and how was your experience at the clinic?

I think I was about 44. I mainly went to the clinic because, at this point, I wanted to check out my health because I had never been pregnant before. I wanted to know if I could conceive and carry a child and what tests I could do and what my next steps could be. Boy, was I in for a rude awakening. Instead of talking about my health, the doctor whipped out a chart from her drawer and showed me a detailed breakdown of possible illnesses a baby could have in relation to the age of the mother—things like developmental disorders, like Down syndrome and other, more severe disorders. I got so scared; I cannot even tell you! She looked at me and said, "At your age of 44, the risks are so high, you should consider an egg donor instead of using your own eggs for fertility treatments."

Now, mind you, I was there to check out my health and to find out if I could conceive naturally, but she just jumped right into the scary risks and the expensive procedures. She told me I could go to their website for twenty-four hours to browse egg donors for free, to see how the system worked and what availability there was for eggs, before committing to the process. All of a sudden, we were talking about the different options of reproductive treatments and the different pricing options. We talked pricing and payment plans, and I realized what a big business it was. These clinics make a fortune from women like me, confronting us with the scary statistics and then immediately leading us down the road of treatment options.

It was overwhelming, and I also had to consider what this would mean for my relationship with Arnoux. I think it would have been the end of our relationship because he is pretty conservative, culturally speaking, and the whole idea of an egg donor and possibly a sperm donor would not have been something he could have supported. There was so much to think about.

As overwhelming as my visit with the fertility clinic was, there was also one very positive aspect to it: I now knew my options, and I felt a bit empowered. It was good to know I had choices, and I think I even scheduled some procedures, which I never followed through with. I knew that I had options if I wanted to bear a child.

And I knew I could adopt. I myself am adopted, and after having me, my mom went on to have two biological children because she felt comfortable again and relaxed. I grew up with this narrative in my mind, that when you prepare emotionally, the physical part will happen. I believe that the unconscious psychological process leads to the physical process. In the end, I did not even have to choose any of these options. I got pregnant naturally at age 45. Arnoux was 60, I think. I call Eden my little miracle.

That's great! How did the father-to-be hold up? Was he in need of an oxygen tent?

I remember the day we found out. I had cramps and went to buy a pregnancy test after work, wondering what in the world I was doing. It was almost like a childhood fantasy, completely magical thinking to believe it could possibly be true. So, I went home and did the test and couldn't believe my eyes. I immediately called Arnoux. He thought I was joking. But he still came over after work and looked at the test himself. Then I called a good friend in New York who is a doctor. Well, he is a psychiatrist, but still *(laughs)*. I told my parents; I called other friends—I was so excited.

Arnoux, on the other hand, was shocked. He was in shock pretty much through the entire pregnancy, which is sad because I was so happy and excited, and I could not really share this excitement with him. In fact, his attitude put a damper on my enthusiasm. We had some stressful moments. When we now speak about that time, he says that he was really scared, mainly because he was focused on the possibility of the baby not being healthy.

His fear led to some intensely negative moments. Before I was ready to share the news with his children, he had told them, and he had shared his anxiety. One of his sons sent a pretty disheartening text to my phone one day—something about being older and all the problems that can come with later motherhood and that I needed to seriously consider all the potential risks. I remember being disgusted and sad. I was aware of the risks and did not need any more fears brought upon me. It made me feel unloved and unsupported.

I am very sorry to hear that, as I remember how vulnerable one feels when pregnant. Physically your pregnancy was good though?

Thankfully, the pregnancy itself was easy, and I felt great. I chose a hospital that had two maternal fetal specialists, just in case. When I went for my first check-up, I was a bit nervous, being 45 and all. I remember the receptionist. She had blonde hair and a lot of makeup—she was so sweet to me. I think I was a bit tearful, a bit emotional about something age-related—I mentioned I am an emotional person, right?—and she just looked at me and said, "Don't worry; we've got a lot of older women here. As a matter of fact, you're really kind of young!" Needless to say, I liked her and the medical team from the start.

There was one hiccup. I had the genetic testing, and the lab test came back with an elevated protein. The doctor told me that we just needed to do the test again and that it was most likely nothing and that I should *not* go onto the internet and read about Spina Bifida, etc. But, of course, that's exactly what I did. I was distraught and called Arnoux, and these were the times when he was supportive and strong. It all turned out well, and Eden is as healthy as they come.

The birth itself was okay. I was low on placenta fluid at the end of the pregnancy, and the doctor admitted me and induced my labor. Unfortunately, I never dilated enough, and when I spiked a fever after twenty-four hours, I had a C-section. This part saddens me a bit, because even though I was afraid of the pain of a vaginal delivery, I wonder how it would have been.

Because of the C-section, they took Eden away so that they could administer antibiotics—I couldn't hold him until after an hour or so of his birth. And he had to stay in the neonatal intensive care unit for two or three days, which messed up our breastfeeding. Since the milk didn't come in as strong, I needed to pump, and things got complicated because of that. But the first moment I was finally able to hold him, it was like Christmas morning, just a thousand times better! As for Arnoux, I think it took him a few months to truly embrace new fatherhood. But now he immensely enjoys being a dad again, and he loves his son and the experience of raising another little boy.

Do you think the fifteen-year age difference between the two of you and the different cultures you grew up in show up in the way you two are parenting?

Yes. When it comes to childcare, I am definitely shouldering the majority of it. Arnoux is not as involved in the day-to-day routine as much as other, younger fathers seem to be. That makes it harder for me, and I am rather tired. In hindsight, I must also say that it was incredibly naïve for me to think that I could have done this alone. Bottom line is that I am grateful for having a partner in raising our child, even though I may be shouldering the majority of work.

Any thoughts about a second child?

I would love to, but at this point, I am too concerned about age-related diseases. I am pro-choice, but personally, I could not consider an abortion if the genetic testing would show an abnormality in the fetus. It makes me sad that Eden will not have a sibling because I think he would very much enjoy that. I am also sad that I did not have him earlier because if I was younger now, I would consider a second child. The upside is that he has extended family in his half-siblings and their kids. Our 2-year-old Eden is uncle to a 12, 9, and 6-year-old, which, one day soon, he will find to be pretty cool.

CHAPTER 13

Claudia S.

Months before I even had my son, a mama in her 40s made my ears perk up. I was listening to Dr. Christiane Northrup on her Hay House radio show, *Flourish*, when she had fertility coach and author Claudia Spahr on as a guest. The two women spoke eloquently about the fear and confusion around later motherhood, and Claudia, who had birthed all three of her naturally conceived children in her 40s, shared tons of solid advice about conception and pregnancy, as well as new data that she had researched for her own book, *Right Time Baby*.

Claudia, a former journalist-turned-author and fertility expert who now resides in Switzerland and Spain, expressed herself with the kind of competence that results from living what she's teaching. While listening to Claudia talk, I looked at her website and saw photos of a slender woman with dark, flowing hair, who looked at least ten years younger than what Dr. Northrup's introduction had suggested. No way this woman was 45—*I want what she's having!*

A couple of weeks later, Claudia and I met for a fun Skype interview during which we talked about becoming moms in our 40s, a conversation journalist to journalist and mom-to-be to new mom of a 4-week-old baby girl. I liked Claudia from the start. Her down-to-earth attitude, solid knowledge of the topic, and easygoing manner—she was rocking her newborn on her lap all during our interview, while occasionally shouting through the open window to her husband who was corralling their two little boys in the yard of their house in Ibiza, Spain—were inspiring. (Watch excerpts of our interview here: *BettinaGordon. com/Bonus*.)

When I reached out to Claudia for this book a couple of years later, we jumped right in. She told me, "I had a string of dysfunctional relationships in my 20s and 30s with men whose sense of family, responsibility, and commitment were practically adolescent. I thought I was 'ready' to become a mom in my early 30s, but with no suitable father candidate around, I threw myself into my career."

For over a decade, Claudia was working in the fast-paced world of television news, racing around with microphones and cameras. For a couple of years, she was the UK correspondent for Swiss TV, which was based in London. It was a highly fascinating job, but it also meant that she was constantly on call and had to drop any personal commitments at a moment's notice—something which is far from ideal if you're a mom. Even though I chose Claudia's interview for the BODY section of this book, you'll see how beautifully all three components of pregnancy—the MIND, the BODY, and the SPIRIT—are interwoven in her story.

Claudia: I changed my lifestyle in my mid-30s to focus on writing. I met my now husband on a trip to India. He was very different than other men I had been with because he really wanted children. But then you could say, maybe I had to change first to attract that kind of man into my life. To be very honest, I just wasn't properly ready to give up my independence or freedom any earlier.

Another interesting point is that my partner is fifteen years younger than me, so he grew up with different gender expectations. I realized early on that he was evolved enough to want to share the job of rearing kids. You could say I met the right man at the right time, which happened to be in my late 30s. Three children later, I am passionate about motherhood at the right time for *you,* the individual woman, not for anybody else.

My mission with my work today is to empower women and to tell them what I believe the real story is and not feed into the fear and confusion that is out there. For women who are trying to conceive, it's really important that they have confidence in their own body and their body's nature and that they be grounded and solid—which is not easy to do when health care providers, the media, and the latest "facts" take away our confidence.

Bettina: How did you become confident yourself?

Well, at first my own experience was that of extreme self-doubt as to whether I would be capable of getting pregnant. That's why I know so well what I am talking about and what so many other women experience. I was rapidly approaching 40, which is a dreaded cultural portal for many women. So many of us think that everything is going to change the moment we hit 40, which, of course, is not true unless your mind is thinking it, which is a very important aspect. But unlike other women who had never been pregnant before, I had already lost a baby. I had just miscarried, and I was getting very impatient and frustrated. Every time I ovulated, I would think about a new beginning, a new chance, and every time I started bleeding again, I'd initially think it was implantation spots, until I realized that this was, indeed, menstrual bleeding. It was disheartening. And I kept having really short periods because my body was just all over the place.

In Chinese medicine, they say that a miscarriage is like a pregnancy and that a woman should give her body time to recover and heal, which is why I now completely understand the dilemma of many women who are going through IVF. They are often rushed to go from one round to the next, to the next, and they mentally feel that there is a time bomb ticking because they will be 40 or 42 or 44, and they cannot possibly lose another month. But what this rush means is that their bodies respond less and less. Our bodies are not machines. The more we try to push them, the less they are able to favorably respond.

A friend of mine said exactly that: "My body is a machine that was not working well. When my car is not working well, I take it to the mechanic. So, when my body was not working well, I took it to a fertility specialist." She had exactly this mindset that you described: my body is a machine, it

is broken, and I need to fix it. My friend pushed and pushed and ended up losing five IVF pregnancies.

Our bodies are not machines that work disconnected from our emotions, thoughts, lifestyle, or belief system. I understand this deeply, as I, too, did not give myself time to heal at first. I wanted to push on. So, I got myself into a place of fear and panic and, yes, desperation, thinking that I had missed my opportunities.

So, what changed?

I had a spiritual experience, which helped me let go, and I believe it opened the door to me getting pregnant with my first child the same month. I was invited to a family constellation session (an alternative therapeutic method) where some issues around guilt and shame came up. They were related to a fear I had about not being worthy of becoming a mother. After acknowledging the fears and forgiving myself, I was able to let go. The therapist showed me a different perspective.

This took me out of my limiting mindset and gave me my confidence back. She also said, "It's going to be fine," and I felt, "Whew, everything is going to be okay." I think she connected with my intuition and was able to mirror it back. It was like instant healing. I'm a rational person but also a spiritual person. Since I'm familiar with yoga and try to practice regularly, I do believe there is more to life than what meets the eye. I think what happens when you have encounters with people who are working with other dimensions is that they perceive more than our limited capacity does. It was very liberating.

This spiritual experience enabled you to leave the fear and doubt behind and trust again?

Yes. I think what happened was that I stopped putting a timer on when I would conceive. I became of the mindset, "It's going to happen when it is going to happen." It was not my interaction with this woman alone that made me regroup—there was something else happening at the same time as well. At the time, my husband and I were living in Ibiza, Spain. One day I was lying by the sea, and all of a sudden, I had the very real and strong feeling that there was a baby around me, a spirit baby. This was not a hallucination; it was a very real feeling.

After this experience, I started reading the book *Spirit Babies* (more about this concept in the SPIRIT pillar) and listened to interviews by a Chinese medicine expert who ran a huge clinic in Houston, Texas, and who, very successfully, had helped women to conceive. She said, and I am paraphrasing, "On the other side, there isn't the same notion of time. If a baby is going to come, it is going to come whether it's this year or next year or in two years. If you are of the mindset that it has to happen now, you may be hindering things, as this mindset is going to cause your body to tense up, and the stress will imbalance your hormones. There is a correlation between stress and not getting pregnant." This made sense to me, and I stopped putting a timer on my pregnancy. As I said, my first son was conceived shortly thereafter.

I've heard many women speak about this and wonder if you believe it too: do you think that there is a divine connection between mother and child, that the soul of the child is connected to the soul of the mother, even before the child is conceived?

Yes, absolutely. I believe in karma and divine connections, and I believe that we have the child that was meant for us. I also think this is true for a miscarriage or abortion. These experiences are part of a soul's journey, and the mother and child are fulfilling something. A miscarriage or an abortion is not necessarily a bad thing; we just don't know what agreement our souls had with the souls of our children. This thought, this belief, was very healing for me and brought me peace in dealing with my own miscarriage.

I kind of believe that things are the way they are meant to be, which is not necessarily what someone who is not able to get pregnant wants to hear. I do think that we have the children we are meant to have—or not. And that includes adoptive children as well. In the book *Spirit Babies*, there is a whole chapter on adoption, and the author describes how two souls, the child and the parent, finally come together through adoption and are no longer separated.

I, too, read the book *Spirit Babies*. When I was pregnant, I was convinced I was having a girl. When we found out we were having a boy, I cried for two days. I still feel a loss for my girl, and I mourn her. I know that may sound really strange because I have this healthy, strong, and beautiful son, whom I enjoy tremendously, and yet I still mourn my daughter as well. And so sometimes I lie down in bed talking to her. I tell her "to find me" and "to come to me." Maybe she will be conceived by another woman and be born through another woman, but maybe, somehow, we will still find each other and be reunited. That's how strongly I feel about her.

I think adoption is really beautiful. My own father was adopted. I believe people often don't understand how deep the bond and connection between a child and the adoptive parent can be.

Did you have a divine experience with your second child as well?

My experience with my second child was different, but there was a divine component as well. In 2010, my husband and I were living for six months in Europe and for six months in South Goa, India. I started to work on my book, *Right Time Baby*, and researched all about later motherhood. I found really encouraging data as well as fertility experts who basically said that pregnancy in your 40s is much more natural than the stories we read would imply. So, I was in a very positive mindset.

I was interested in having another baby, but at the time, my husband was not so inclined. I also went to see my gynecologist for a check-up, and he found a very big cyst on one of my ovaries, which apparently can happen to women when they stop breastfeeding. He said we should keep a close eye on the cyst as it can become dangerous and may have to be surgically removed. Oh, and this cyst would keep me from getting pregnant. So, I thought, "Gosh, no, I have no pain. I don't want to have an operation! I'd rather find other ways to heal my body!"

Oh, by the way, I see a huge focus on women being healthy and living a clean life before they conceive, but men are often left out of the equation. This is a big error as men's sperm count and quality has gone down dramatically in the last few decades. I wrote about it in my book, *Right Time Baby*. Industrialized farming affected the men who worked in this industry really negatively.

When you ask the fertility specialists, you actually find out that 40 to 50 percent of the time it's the man who has fertility issues, not the woman. The sperm is not as healthy as it used to be, and that makes it harder for women to conceive healthy children. Just recently I was listening to an Australian fertility expert who talked about new research that said that the egg compensates for any damage in the DNA of the sperm. So, if there is damage in the DNA of a sperm, the egg has to work so much harder to create an embryo.

Often, we think that miscarriage is the women's "fault," while it may be that the sperm could not produce a healthy embryo that was growing properly. It can get a bit tricky for some women to convince their partners to have their sperm checked as the guys often think of themselves as infallible. But checking out the quality of the sperm should be one of the first things a couple does. And then the couple can get into a healthier lifestyle together.

Shortly after my doctor's visit, my husband and I left for South Goa and lived close to the beach. The news about the cyst encouraged me to do a detox and to practice yoga on a regular basis. We both ate healthy vegetarian food and observed our circadian rhythm. We were not exposed to computers at night or to TV, and we were very grounded. Through yoga, my body became stronger, and I felt strong and healthy and very vital. I felt confident in my body.

So here we are back with the body confidence piece you mentioned earlier.

Yes. I was strong and confident, and I think I was also letting go of any expectation or sense of time. I was just in the here and now, feeling strong but not focusing on getting pregnant. If it's meant to happen, it will happen—I am not even going to think about it. It was a very subtle shift.

Since my husband did not want to have another child, we were careful not to get pregnant. However, one time we didn't pay attention, and I got pregnant immediately. The cyst did not matter; the fact that my husband was not so sure about a second child did not matter. It happened anyway. It was really like a one-hit wonder! It's interesting, but for many women I talk to who got pregnant in their 40s, or even 50s, it happened like this. They stopped taking precautions and got pregnant from having unprotected intercourse—all it took was just that one time.

I think it's also a sign that, when the spirit baby is ready to come in and you are relaxed about pregnancy in body, mind, and spirit, there only needs to be a small window of opportunity. I truly believe what the author of *Spirit Babies* writes: "When a soul wants to come in, it will come in no matter what!" It actually also happened to us again in getting pregnant with our daughter, our third child. I was 44 at the time, and I know exactly when she was conceived. I even joked afterwards, "Oh, don't worry; you know what they say about the chances at my age." So much for listening to mainstream advice.

Are you up for child number four?

I love having children, but I feel called to do other things now. I just turned 47, and I often forget how old I even am. I am totally sure that I could easily get pregnant again. So, my answer is that I think we are done, but we are still careful.

CHAPTER 14

BODY Action Steps

Chronological Versus Biological Age

You have read it before in this book: your chronological age (the age on your driver's license) and your biological age (the age of your body) are not necessarily the same. In fact, they can be disparately different. At age 44, Sara Gottfried, the Harvard- and MIT-educated physician and bestselling author I mentioned before, decided that she wanted to know the truth about her biological age, something which can be measured in a person's blood by way of a test for telomere length. Telomeres are caps on your chromosomes that show how quickly you are aging on a cellular and biological level, as opposed to chronological one. The cells in your body have telomeres, and each time a cell divides, its telomeres get shorter. It's normal to lose telomere length as you age, but only at a certain, healthy rate.

Well, Dr. Sara was in for quite a surprise: "My telomeres were as short and stubby as the ones of a 64-year-old! Here I was, a board-certified doctor in gynecology, and I did not know that the stress hormone cortisol had been shrinking my telomeres, increasing my risk for cancer as well as such things as more belly fat and diabetes. I had not been aware of the toll the stressful years of residency or the sleep deprivation from having two children had taken on my body or that it had accelerated my aging."

Dr. Sarah, also known for her expertise in women's hormonal health, set out on a journey and searched for all the "levers for growing younger" that can slow down and, in her case, quite literally reverse the aging process. She presents her scientific findings in her latest book, *Younger*, which I found to be an exceptionally interesting read. Dr. Sara closed the gap between her chronological and her biological age by seventeen years and now has the telomeres of a 52-year-old, which is only three years older than her current age of 49. Soon she will be chronologically in her 50s, but biologically in her 40s.

You Can Influence Your Health and Biological Age

This chapter is actually doubly important to us grown-up women: with the action steps below, we can improve our fertility *and* our biological age, which will come in handy when we chase little ones through the house in our 40s and 50s or deal with teenagers when we hit our 60s (which will be me—Hunter will be 16 when I hit 60. Gulp. My telomeres better be long and lean by then). And it hopefully gives you added incentive to follow through with your "fertility rejuvenation," as Oriental medicine expert Aimee Raupp puts it.

Reports published in the renowned scientific journal *Obstetrics & Gynecology* suggest that mere lifestyle and diet modification can improve the chances of conception in 80 percent of the females above 40 who lack a gross systemic or organic issue that is interfering with getting pregnant. So, if your doctor tells you that diet and lifestyle changes cannot improve fertility, please consider switching your doctor immediately, as she does not read up on the current scientific findings.

Full disclosure: I used to roll my eyes when somebody told me about the toxins in our food and our environment, the dangers of genetically modified foods, or the dreadful impact of plastics on our health. I thought it was just fear mongering and that federal agencies, like the Food and Drug Administration or the Environmental Protection Agency, had strong, unbiased laws in place to keep us safe. (Okay, that assumption was naïve on my part.) Then I did my research for this book. And now I take this matter very seriously. You and I, we cannot rely on public agencies and authority figures to tell us what is safe to consume and use—we need to use our own judgment and research and be our own advocate, especially advocating for our children's health and future. Once you peak behind the curtain, you'll be shocked by what you find. I will certainly be writing more about this topic in the years to come.

I also want you to please view this chapter not just as "suggestions" or things to dabble in but as hard facts and solid evidence that will improve your overall health and thus enhance your fertility. In an ideal world, we'd do all the steps suggested in this chapter to make the biggest positive impact, and I salute you if you do. But I also understand that this list may seem daunting, maybe even overwhelming, to some of us. Please don't get stressed about all the things you *should* do but eventually won't do because the task seems too big. This is not an all-or-nothing approach. If this list is too daunting, pick a few areas where you see the most room for improvement and do those. Every action taken will lead to better health. You *can* do it!

As previously discussed, take at least three months—or, even better, six to nine months—to follow the actions steps below. Why that long? First: only a healthy egg can create a healthy baby. The cycle of an egg in preparation for ovulation (when the egg is released and travels down the fallopian tube where it may be met by a sperm and become fertilized) is around ninety days. During these ninety days, before an egg reaches full maturation, it is affected by both healthy and unhealthy influences, like hormonal balance, nutritional intake, or stress. By observing a healthy and fertility-focused lifestyle for a minimum of three months, you can boost the health of your egg. Second: ideally, you want to cleanse and nourish your body, and thus enhance your egg quality, for longer than just three months—after years, possibly decades, of ill treatment, your miraculous body may need more time to heal and fully recover. Better err on the side of caution.

And remember Dr. Sara's 90/10 rule from the BODY introduction chapter: only 10 percent of our risks for disease come from our genes—90 percent is lifestyle and environment. Our health is 90 percent in our hands, and it's the daily choices we make and the dedication we show that determines our health's fate, whether we become moms or not.

Stop Hindering Your Fertility

The term "too old" for a baby does not necessarily refer to age but to hormone status. In menopause, our natural hormone levels are too low to support a pregnancy. The timing of menopause, though, is largely determined by the amount of toxins in our bodies and the lack of vitamins and minerals, as this accelerates the aging process. So, let's do something about this, as effectively as possible.

According to *foodrevolution.org*, there are more than eighty-thousand chemicals in widespread use in America *per day*, and they are found in the food we eat, in the products we use, in the water we drink, and in the air we breathe. Since our own childhood, the exposure to harmful toxins in our environment has skyrocketed, and you can find study after study confirming the dangers we are exposed to and the harmful effects they have on our health and, thus, our fertility. Thankfully we can all take powerful measures to protect ourselves from further harm and to rid our bodies of pollution.

Out with the Bad

Go through your personal care items and throw out or donate any conventional product you put on your skin (which is your body's largest organ and can absorb most of the chemicals) and scalp, including your body lotion and hair care products, especially if you use them on a daily basis. Also include your toothpaste, your sun lotion, nail polish, and your detergent. Toss the bleach and fabric softener.

This may seem radical, yes, but if you know that personal care products are manufactured with 10,500 unique chemical ingredients, some of which are known or suspected carcinogens, toxic to the reproductive system, or known to disrupt the endocrine system, you may rethink your beauty regimen. FYI: the American government doesn't require health studies or pre-market testing of the chemicals in personal care products, even though just about everyone is exposed to them (*check out http://www.ewg.org/skindeep/myths-on-cosmetics-safety/*).

Of course, your nail polish or shampoo alone will not jeopardize the health of your baby, but because we've used these products in combination for decades, often daily, the toxins have accumulated in our bodies, and it's time for a radical clean up. Should you be too attached to your beauty products to throw them out, then put them in a box out of reach and replace them with safe products for the pre-conception phase, all through the pregnancy, and through the time you are breastfeeding. That you can do for sure.

In with the Good

To replace your personal care products, go to *http://www.ewg.org/skindeep/* and check out the Environmental Working Group's database for healthy and safe products. Personally, I use organic coconut oil ($4.99 for sixteen ounces at ALDI supermarket) as body lotion for myself and for my child, and I use the same organic coconut oil (different jar) for cooking. I'll always remember what my late friend Horst Rechelbacher, the founder of the natural cosmetic chain Aveda—now owned by Estee Lauder—and Intelligent Nutrients, a company that produces hair and skin care that is certified (!) organic, once said to me: "You should not put anything on your skin that you could not also drink!" He offered me a bottle of shampoo to taste—I smiled and declined. I got the point. Since then, I've used the Intelligent Nutrient products myself.

No More Plastic, Thank You Very Much

Stop drinking unfiltered tap water and bottled water. Retire all your plastic containers, as harmful substances such as bisphenol A (BPA), bisphenol S (BPS), and bisphenol F (BPF) leach into water and any food you might store in them. I am always perplexed to see single fruits or vegetables wrapped in plastic foil in the supermarkets or apples encased in big plastic trays. This is not only a huge waste of plastic and a burden on the environment (in the landfill, plastic components take up to one-thousand years to break down, all the while leaching into the ground and polluting groundwater reservoirs), but they are also dangerous to our health and to the health of our children in utero. BPA and phthalates, found in food packaging and medical devices are, according to *Environment Health News*, present in 90 percent of premature babies. Do these chemicals cause premature births? I don't know, but I wonder about the connection.

Go through your cleaning supplies and find less-toxic options. Throw out scented candles, air fresheners, and basically everything that makes the air inside your house "smell good" by emitting chemicals. The Environmental Working Group has a safety rating for more than 2,500 products right here: http://www. ewg.org/guides/cleaners.

Clean Water Is Key

Invest in a high-end water filter (my husband brought his beloved filter into our marriage) that attaches to the faucet or is installed underneath the sink, such as a Reverse Osmosis System. Reuse glass bottles for your drinking water and store all food items in glass containers as well. Drinking lots of clean water is important for you, and clean water will be especially important when your child is born, as little bodies get polluted quickly (for more articles on how to shield your child from harmful substances, please check out my website *BettinaGordon. com*).

You Are Investing in Your and Your Baby's Health

If you are concerned about the costs of your product makeover, please look at this as an investment in your health that will save you in medical bills later in life. And if these suggestions seem a bit over the top at first, just know that, by taking a radical step (or multiple baby steps) today, you will also protect the health of your baby in utero.

In 2005 a study that was spearheaded by the Environmental Working Group found, on average, 200 industrial chemicals and pollutants in umbilical cord blood of babies born in the United States the previous summer. The umbilical cord blood of these children harbored pesticides, consumer product ingredients, and industrial chemicals and waste. Of the 287 chemicals detected, 180 cause cancer in humans or animals, 217 are toxic to the brain and nervous system, and 208 cause birth defects or abnormal development in animal tests. We hope the dangers of pre- or post-natal exposure to this complex mixture of carcinogens, developmental toxins, and neurotoxins will soon be properly studied.

The point is this: your baby may not only inherit your good looks but also a chemical cocktail in your womb that could affect his health.

Know Your Body, Know Your Hormones

Many of the chemicals and toxins in our environment are so-called endocrine disrupters, which means that they not only pollute our bodies but also interfere with our hormones and our bodies' ability to function as they should. For example, endocrine disruptors can artificially raise your estrogen levels, and having a high level of estrogen can prevent conception through the creation of PCOS and endometriosis. Hormones like estrogen, progesterone, FSH, or thyroid stimulating hormone (TSH) play a key role in fertility. The good news is that you can affect your hormones naturally; however, if your doctor does not tell you this (maybe he does not even know), you may look at your blood test and be devastated by a low FSH, thinking you only have a 5 to 8 percent chance to naturally conceive (as was Denise's experience, chapter 11).

It is utterly important for us women to know how our endocrine system works and what we can do to naturally boost (or lower) the levels of certain hormones to increase our fertility and keep a pregnancy once it occurs. Knowledge is key here. But do we have it?

The female body is a miraculous work of art, in which every organ, every gland, and every cell has a function to fulfill. Do you know how our female organs work? Do you know about the four phases of our menstrual cycle? Did you ever experience symptoms like heavy bleeding, irregular periods, or cramps? Were you taught how to bring your hormones back to balance, or did your doctor offer to put you on the pill to manage your symptoms?

It really is not our fault that we women often don't know what's really going on with our bodies and our hormonal health. Cue in fertility experts like Alisa Vitti to become the teachers we never had. There are many good books on the market about hormonal health (Dr. Sara Gottfried wrote two of these, for example), yet I found Alisa's book *WomanCode* to be especially interesting because she puts a big focus on fertility and tells you not only what to do but also why to do it. If you are anything like me, the "why" is vital.

Alisa's Five-Step Protocol is designed to address the underlying cause of hormonal problems and to support the essential functions of your endocrine system so your hormones can work in a healthy and balanced way. The steps are 1) stabilize your blood sugar; 2) nurture your adrenal glands; 3) support your organs of elimination; 4) sync with your menstrual cycle; 5) engage your feminine energy. Whatever you decide to do, this is a good framework to consider, and I recommend reading *WomanCode* to understand your body and your hormonal health. In addition, please listen to my interview with Alisa in the resource membership area to gain a better grasp of this topic (*BettinaGordon.com/Bonus*).

Detoxify Your Body

Let's clean out the toxins that have already accumulated in your body with a cleanse that actually supports your fertility. This will give you extra mileage if you are over 40, as most other women don't think about detoxifying their bodies, let alone do it. (Important note: do *not* detox once you are pregnant because the released toxins would go straight into the baby through the umbilical cord.) A fertility cleanse focuses on two specific organs: the liver and the uterus. Why the liver? The main job of the liver is to filter out the toxins in the body and get rid of excess hormones. If there is an excess of estrogen, the liver needs extra help to dispel the hormone, something you can do by using herbs and supplements (that's what I did). And uterine health is super important for fertility, of course.

Every cycle, the uterus is supposed to release the lining that had built up that month for any potential embryo to implant. In some cases, the uterus is not completely cleansed every cycle, so old, stagnant blood remains. As you can imagine, this is not the best environment to house a new embryo. Please listen to my interview with Hethir Rodriguez, founder of *Natural Fertility Info*, in which she lays out all the benefits a fertility cleanse has on a woman's body (also found in the membership section). Support your cleanse with the following:

- castor oil packs (applied to your lower abdomen)
- exercise, such as walking or yoga, in general, and fertility yoga, in particular
- fertility massages (that you can also do yourself)

Nourish Your Body from the Inside Out

The foods you eat today impact the quality of the egg and sperm ninety days from now. How is that for a reframe of the word "diet"?!

I cannot stress enough that the choices you make today around food and drink will have real impact on your health and the health of your future child. Our food supply is unfortunately riddled with processed foods, void of nutrients but full of ingredients made in a lab, rather than the earth, and substances made by scientists, rather than chefs. According to the website *Natural Fertility Info*, Americans consume over a pound of pesticides unknowingly each year—yikes!

Since I am passionate about the topic of food and healthy nutrition for myself, but especially for my boy, Hunter, I am on the email list of food activists like *foodrevolution.org, foodbabe.com, fooddemocracynow.org*, and *fmtv.com* and others, and I get the news right in my inbox. The highest amount of weed killer residue found in popular food? Children's Cheerios. One of the unhealthiest food choices today? Farmed fish. Which most-beloved fruit should children never eat unless it's organic? Strawberries.

Your fertility is closely linked to your food and drink choices, and the preconception phase is as crucial for you and your child as the nine months of pregnancy, when your body builds a whole human out of one particular cell. Think not of food as "diet" but rather as "medicine" and put the health of your child before your food temptations. That was my biggest motivator—I tend to let things slide much more easily when it's only about me. But if it's about my kid, boy, I can easily muster the stamina to say no to frozen pizza and packaged pasta. (Okay, relatively easily.)

Here it is in a nutshell: nature has created food that nourishes and feeds the body, and that's what we should consume. Stay away from highly processed and prepackaged foods. Avoid fruit juices and sugar. Ditch the soda and alcohol. If your grandmother would not have recognized a food as food, don't consume it. Eat a lot of organic vegetables and fruits. Consume only free-range organic chicken and organic and grass-fed meats. Be very picky with fish and go for cold-water varieties. Go for lots of dark, leafy greens. Drink filtered water. Use high-quality fats like olive oil, sesame oil, and, for high-heat cooking, coconut oil and ghee. If your body already deals with chronic inflammation (like mine), the natural fertility experts recommend cutting out gluten, sugar, soy, and dairy.

Virtually every natural fertility expert I spoke to had a strong focus on nutrition and diet. Alisa Vitti created a protocol of fertility-boosting foods to consume during the four phases of your menstrual cycle (which are called the follicular, ovulatory, luteal, and menstrual phases, by the way), while Aimee Raupp will put you on her fertility rejuvenation protocol. As I mentioned before, if you can, consider joining a program that firmly catapults you onto a healthy path so you can try to conceive more quickly than if you went at it alone. In terms of health, we have no time to waste. You can find helpful resources and tips at *BettinaGordon.com/Bonus.*

America Runs on Dunkin—but Not If You'd Like to Get Pregnant

One big point to make here: keep blood sugar stable, starting from the time you wake up. When insulin (a hormone) levels are erratic, it suppresses ovulation. The worst thing you can do when you want to get pregnant is have a cup of coffee on an empty stomach. (I know. I almost spit out my cafe latte when I first heard this on a webinar.)

Your blood sugar has been low after a night's rest, and by spiking it with coffee, you set up your insulin levels to fluctuate erratically for the rest of the day and disturb your ovulation for the entire cycle. The newest research by the American College of Obstetric Oncology has found that caffeine consumption increases miscarriage rates. Caffeine is so powerful that even if you don't drink any but your husband is a heavy coffee drinker, it can affect your ability to conceive.

Boost Your Vitamin and Mineral Storage

If you have looked into natural ways to boost your fertility, you already know that vitamin D is important and that royal jelly and Maca root have the reputation of being fertility superfoods. Since I am not an herbalist, I'd like to send you over to Hethir Rodriguez.. You will find a lot of high-quality, research-based information on her site *Natural Fertility Info*.

The next three tips come from one of my favorite experts in women's health: Yale-educated MD, Aviva Romm (also a midwife and herbalist for three decades).

Get to Your Optimal Weight

This is not just a matter of vanity. Women who enter pregnancy overweight have a much higher risk of prenatal and birth complications and a much higher chance of needing a C-section. The baby is much more likely to have a host of health problems, ranging from allergies, asthma, and obesity in childhood to diabetes and heart disease later in life. Find the right program for you, based on whole foods, wise eating habits, and yoga or some other fave form of exercise. Having the body you love now could help you have the healthiest baby possible down the road.

De-Stress

Stress messes with your hormones and causes fertility problems. It messes with your blood sugar and insulin levels and causes pregnancy problems. And stress in pregnancy can lead to depression, anxiety, and obesity in our kids. In fact, it's estimated that at least 80 percent of all health problems are caused by stress. Wowza! That's a lot of mess from stress. Okay, some stress is unavoidable—but the goal here is to keep it from hijacking your life.

So, pick your healing tool: yoga, meditation, exercise, counseling, making scary but needed life/work/relationship transformations . . . just do it. Conquer that stress and cultivate peace. This equals a better you, better babies, and a better world.

Have the Guts to Protect the Next Generation

Of course, you can't get through an article on a health website these days without hearing about the microbiome. But did you know that a person's gut flora is pretty much determined by age three, and most of it's all thanks to mom? Mom having healthy gut flora (and then having a vaginal birth and breastfeeding) is like investing in gold for baby's gut flora bank account. And it all starts long before pregnancy.

The following list outlines the top things you can do to create a healthy gut flora:

- Avoid antibiotics (unless, of course, they're truly necessary—and they rarely are).
- Eat a wide variety of foods, especially leafy greens and fermented foods.
- Take a good-quality probiotic.

Know Your Fertile Time but Have Sex Twice a Week, Every Week

There is a lot of free information available about the right time to have intercourse in order to conceive. Personally, I bought the classic *Taking Charge of Your Fertility* by Toni Weschler and found all the information I needed in order to read my body's fertile signs without having to chart. Please do the research yourself to find the method that suits you best. I'd like to point out something here that is at least as important as the relationship you will have with your child and that is having a loving and strong relationship with the partner you will have your child with.

Timing sex with ovulation can be stressful and often reduces lovemaking to a sexual chore. Friends of mine had struggled to conceive for quite some time. Then, finally, the long-awaited son was born. Three years later, my friends got divorced. "We never found our way back again to the connection we had before we tried to conceive," both acknowledged later on. Their intimate sexual bond was lost, and eventually their whole relationship deteriorated. That's why I love Aimee Raupp's suggestion to her clients: have sex twice a week every week with your partner. Keep the intimate bond strong, especially during trying times (pun intended), and know that a woman's body becomes more fertile the more sex she has. I'm sure your partner will happily oblige.

CHAPTER 15

Pillar Three: SPIRIT

You and Your Baby

In June of 2013, I took a gondola up to the top of one of Italy's highest Alpine ranges, the legendary Dolomites. There, in a one-hundred-year-old hut that had a breathtaking view of the mountains from a weathered, wooden window, I took my pregnancy test and carefully put it on the edge of the sink. It was a pretty surreal moment for me. When I saw the two blue lines appear, I dashed out and ran straight to my friend Brigitte. Since Joshua was still in the United States and not scheduled to arrive in Europe for another ten days, I was so happy to have her there. Brigitte is a smart and successful business lady who happened to be madly in love with her two kids. It had been so inspiring for me to see how she valued her children and unabashedly made them her priority while still rocking her business.

Brigitte and I laughed and hugged and jumped up and down like teenagers. I literally got high on the endorphins (the "feel-good" hormones) that were rushing through my body. We took pictures, and I recorded a video for my baby right there, on top of the mountain, with the clear blue sky spanning like a dome above me (check out the photos of this magical place in the travel section of my website). All of a sudden, two female hikers appeared next to us. One carried a big belly in front of her and smiled at me. She was almost eight months pregnant and still hiking with joy. I took her appearance as a very fortuitous sign. To say I was elated is a gross understatement.

Then I did what I felt like I needed to do: I walked away and found a quiet place to sit by a tree and stare at the panorama. As I rested my back against the tree trunk, I went quiet and started listening for any small voice inside me that potentially had doubts about this pregnancy. I had been so ambivalent and torn about motherhood for so many years that I needed to check in with myself to see if this positive pregnancy test was indeed just positive or if I still had doubts that I was doing the right thing. Being up on the mountain and realizing that all my concerns had vanished was a profound spiritual experience for me. It was divine in the truest sense of the word.

(On our way down the mountain, we crossed many pastures full of free-roaming goats, sheep, and cows. At one point, we were attacked by a seriously mad cow and had to jump into high bushes for safety. As we dashed away from the 1,600-pound beast, all I could think was, "I just found out I am pregnant—that's really bad timing to be trampled by a cow!" But that's another story.)

One of the biggest advantages of being an older mom is the life experience, the awareness, and the wisdom we can bring to motherhood and offer our children. We have all overcome obstacles and doubts and have grown and matured into who we are today in both our professional and private lives. We have a lot to offer our children—just think back on the last couple of decades and how you evolved from a young teenager to the accomplished and experienced woman you are now. What are the craziest moments of your life? The most rewarding? The most contemplative? The ones that fill you with love? The ones that fill you with pride? The ones that you'd rather forget? The ones you may not want to acknowledge publicly but look back on fondly?

Our rich lives and experiences shape the way we guide our children on their own paths and the life we can provide for them. We will uniquely parent, yet as I found out in my interviews, there are many commonalities that we mature parents seem to share:

- Many of us are highly educated and pursue a (first, second, or third) career we feel aligned with. We tend to be financially stable and well off.
- We often have access to top-level education and health care for our family.
- Many of us have built up clout at work and can negotiate more time with our families.
- We tend to re-evaluate our careers. Quite a few women I spoke to chose to significantly scale back at work or stay at home with their child for a couple of years.
- We have often forged a strong and stable relationship with our partners. At our age, we know that the grass is always greener *until you reach the other side*. Fun fact: a good third of the women I interviewed have partners younger than them (including me). Six of them are with men ten to fifteen years their junior.
- We tend to know who we are and what we bring to the table. In all my interviews, I never heard a mom say, "I lost myself after becoming a mother."
- We are less concerned and frazzled about the small stuff. We have learned to see the bigger picture.
- We have overcome many obstacles and developed an "I've got this" attitude.
- We are health conscious and are, in general, mindful about the food we give our children.
- We tend to worry that our time with our kids will be cut short. Staying healthy and active is a priority for us.
- We often have only one child and are concerned about that. Some of us wish we would have had our child sooner so there would have been enough time and energy for a second one.
- About a third of the women I interviewed felt a lack of energy as they got older.
- If we were big travelers before having kids, we will take them with us on the road and give them admission to a bigger world.

- We appreciate and indulge in time with our children, as we have no FOMO, no fear of missing out. Party all night? Been there, done that. Bath and bedtime reading with the kids, no high heels required? Sign me up!
- From time to time, many of us struggle with the loss of freedom and independence that we've fostered for decades. And we long for quiet times on the couch, coffee or drink and newspaper in hand.
- We hire the nannies and au pairs that give us freedom and time when we need them. As I like to say, "Childcare is health care."
- We are emotionally and psychologically stable. We yell less, impose fewer physical punishments, and tend to encourage our kids more, something which a new Danish study, published in the *European Journal of Development*, confirms.
- We have the awareness of how our own behavior influences that of our children, and we are mindful not to put our "stuff" on them.
- Most of us have the courage to listen to our instincts instead of doing whatever the majority of parents do. We did not succumb to society's pressure to procreate early, and we will not succumb to parent peer pressure now.
- Many of us feel that there is a spiritual side to creating life.

One of the most beautiful and touching findings in my many conversations with the new moms was how often and how eloquently so many women spoke about their faith and trust in a higher power. They expressed their feeling that having a baby was not only up to them and their partners or a medical team. For them, there was another power at play that worked *together* with them, a spiritual partner if you will, whom they recognized and, at some point, surrendered to.

Depending on their personal beliefs and cultural upbringing, the women spoke about their faith in God, a benevolent and loving being who wanted them to have a baby and ultimately gave them the gift of a child. Other women spoke about losing their beloved mother, grandfather, or sister and how they felt that the spirits of their loved ones came back to them when they became pregnant, even if they never really thought about such a possibility before. Some women talked about connecting with the spirit of their future child and how they felt the child's presence, even heard its voice from time to time, before it was even conceived. And, maybe most valuable, they spoke about keeping their faith and their spiritual connection strong even if—or especially when—they experienced miscarriages and emotions of loss or despair.

It all made me realize that there is a profound third pillar to pregnancy (next to the commonly accepted MIND and BODY) that I call SPIRIT, as it relates so strongly to the spirit of the mother and how she navigates her journey to pregnancy and into motherhood. SPIRIT also relates to the spirit of our future children and the spirit of something greater than ourselves, whether you call it God, the universe, or the divine. After dozens of conversations, I saw certain commonalities between these women who found solace and strength in how their worldview started to (re)shape itself once motherhood became what they desired. And it seems that even impending and not just actual pregnancy made them more instinctual and more in tune with their own spirituality.

In general, I noticed a certain progression of events that naturally unfolded for many of the women I spoke to, regardless of whether they considered themselves spiritual or religious or nothing at all. I include these steps in this pillar because rarely is a woman's spirit and soul more tested and more engaged than when she wants to bring forth life.

For this SPIRIT introduction chapter, I decided to introduce concepts that you may have never heard about or contemplated, such as establishing a spiritual connection to your unborn child. For some, the topics discussed may feel like "homecoming," and for others, they may feel "too far out" and difficult to relate to. Spirituality, beliefs, and faith—or the absence thereof—are very personal choices, and you may relate to this chapter enthusiastically or maybe not very much. Even if you are not a spiritually minded person and don't relate to this chapter immediately, I would still invite you to read the interviews, if you'd like, and definitely read the SPIRIT Action Steps, as topics like stress and how to lower its effect on your body or the importance of choosing—yes, choosing—happiness are beneficial for everyone.

I Will Be Okay

One of the toughest starting points for women is when they first feel that they are ready to start their family, but they do not have the man in their life they'd like to do it with. Personally, I know very well how this feels; for ten years in New York City, I was without a significant other. I met Joshua when I was 36 years old, and we got married when I was 38. Being without the right partner is a profoundly challenging situation because, on the one hand, there's hope that he'll eventually show up, but on the other hand, there's fear that, by then, it may be too late and motherhood may never happen.

It takes a lot of guts to still keep hope alive and not give in to the pressure (from outside factors and ourselves) to procreate with a man who is wrong for us. The women whose stories you have already read have dealt with this issue in their own ways, but I also reached out to Lucy Johnson. Lucy is a psychotherapist who works with women who are "circumstantially childless" (not having met the right partner) in her practice in London as well as through Skype. Lucy was 42 and 44 when she, herself, became a mom, and she had some very good advice to share.

Lucy explained to me, "Not having a child when you want one can feel as profoundly upsetting as biological infertility. The question then is: how can I come to terms with where I am now? I encourage my clients to process the fear and grief they feel when they think that motherhood may potentially not happen for them. This can be hard to own up to because, with it, can come a sense of shame, the shame of feeling that we have, in some ways, failed at achieving motherhood. This is made doubly bad by the fact that not only is this type of grief unrecognized by society, but it is also often judged: 'You don't have a man because you are too picky'; 'You are not pregnant because you focused on your career.' Who wants to sit with all of this and feel what comes up inside?

"Many women do feel grief at the loss of an imagined future or a sense of themselves as a mother. But what I find is that, if we unpack these emotions underneath the surface and process them, we can come to some feelings of resolution. We can explore how circumstance has impacted us as women—busy career, the limited pool of suitable men, etc. We can own our feelings, including grief and shame, and transform them into a deeper understanding of ourselves.

And we can take back control from a sense of helplessness by exploring the areas we do have a choice in: Can we create more of a work/life balance? What sort of men are we choosing and why? Are these men father material? And if not, why not? At the end, we cannot know if we will become mothers. Many of us will; some will not. But with my clients I find that, for those who do the deep emotional excavation work and look their potential loss in the face, it can give birth to something else: a new creativity, wisdom, and maturity that enables them to go on and lead joyous and productive lives, whether they become mothers or not."

I've heard it over and over again and have had my own version of it as well: when we walk through the dark night of the soul and have faced our fears, we can and will reach that deep understanding that, regardless of what happens, *we will be okay.* So, regardless of whether we have not met the right partner yet or have gone through miscarriage or are afraid we'll lose the man we love if we cannot get pregnant, this knowing that "whatever comes my way, I will be okay" seems like the first step to taking a bigger, more empowered, and more spiritual view of our roles as potential mothers. It's the foundation, the basis from which everything else flourishes.

Surrender

For those of us who have worked hard to build a professional career and who usually achieve what we set out to achieve, "surrender" is simply not in our vocabularies. We are go-getters, organizers, and reapers of our labor. We like having things under control, and we know that if we do ABC, we most likely will see the desired XYZ outcome. So, once we know what we can do to boost our fertility, we follow the diet, do the yoga, get the acupuncture, and make sure our partners follow their regimen as well. We expect to see the two pregnancy lines on the pregnancy stick as a result of our efforts. I repeat, we expect to see them. Again, we expect to see them—*now!* . . . So, where the hell are they?

"I had everything mapped out and followed my plan to the T," Sasha remembered. "But when I did not get pregnant naturally for a whole year, I was devastated. I was 41 by then, and I had gotten tense and angry at my situation. I felt ashamed and alone, as I don't think even my husband understood what was going on. I mean, I make mountains move at work, but I could get pregnant even once?

"I remember sitting on a bench in New York's Central Park one day, staring at the parents pushing their strollers, and somehow it hit me. I thought, 'What if this is not only up to me? What if God or a higher power or whatever you want to call it also has a say? Oh, f***!' *(laughs)* This knocked me down like a ton of bricks, and the following Sunday, I returned to my church for the first time in years!"

Two years after this event, Sasha and I sat on the bench of her church's courtyard in downtown Manhattan, and tears started streaming down her face as she remembered those days. "Do we really think our lives are in our hands only? That it is only up to us if we will or will not have a baby?"

"What do you think?" I asked.

"Once I embraced that my life is not only up to me, I surrendered. I had grown up Catholic, but had not practiced in decades. I started to pray again. Mind you, I did not give up on my dream of holding my baby, but I surrendered to the divine and to the notion that I did what I could do and now it was time for God to help me. I used to think that surrender is weak, but I realized that it takes an awful lot of courage to let go of control and of the need to be in charge. There was something incredibly liberating and peaceful in my surrender because, for the first time in years, I realized that it would not be my fault alone if I'd never be a mother. The heaviness of conception was no longer squarely on my shoulders, and I found solace in knowing that ultimately my life and my child's life were in God's hands."

After she surrendered, Sasha noticed a shift happening in her attitude, her physical being (she was less tense, less angry, and more at ease with what is), as well as a change in her relationship with her husband. Maybe all these shifts contributed to her pregnancy, or maybe it was truly all in God's hands, but shortly before her 43rd birthday, Sasha finally held her baby daughter in her arms. A little later, amidst trying to breastfeed, sleep, keep the baby clean, and, most important, alive, Sasha again realized she was no longer in control of so much in her life. And to her surprise, she's mostly fine with that. And so are the dozen other women who told me similar stories of surrender.

In their unique way, the majority of women I interviewed had similar stories to share: "I surrounded myself with my nieces and nephews as much as I could to fill up on their love"; "I produced the most amazing pieces of art I had ever done"; "I booked a trip to Galapagos for my husband and me and bought a brand-new camera as I am a passionate photographer." At some point, we realized that living in the *here and now* and actively focusing on what makes us happy was a pivotal choice on our journey.

Tune in and Communicate

During one of my many travels over a decade ago, I joined a revered Native American elder on a ten-day journey through New Mexico and Colorado and learned firsthand some of the ancient rituals Native Americans had been practicing for centuries. This was a truly profound experience. I also distinctively remember standing at the edge of Sun Temple in Colorado's ancient Mesa Verde National Park, with my arms spread wide, feeling the wind rushing through the canyon toward me. The landscape and the energy of Mesa Verde opened me up like none of the remarkable cathedrals of my Roman Catholic upbringing ever had before. My heart blew wide open, and I allowed myself to feel, really feel, instead of having my mind rule the show.

As I stood there at Sun Temple, I viscerally felt in my whole being that my scientific mindset—which I had arrogantly thought made me superior to people of a less scientific, Western-educated worldview—had kept me small. I had followed the old adage "seeing is believing"—what could not be scientifically explained and measured could not exist. At Mesa Verde, I realized there was a whole big world out there that I had never considered before: the world of the unseen, the unexplainable, the unconventional, and "non-rational." (For me, this was different from religion, yet for others, it may be the same.)

Back home in New York City, I started to research intuition and ancient traditions, and for three years, I took part in the profound training at the Women's Ways Mystery School led by my spiritual teacher (believe me, if you had told me back in my 20s that one day I'd have a spiritual teacher, I would have laughed in your face), Lorraine Simone, aka Deep Arrow Woman, in Southampton, New York. After years of deepening my own personal understanding of spirituality, I realized that "seeing is believing" may be an outdated model. *Believing is what lets us see.*

So, when the first woman started to talk to me about her communication with her unconceived child, I did not think it strange. Just because we cannot scientifically prove something to be possible does not mean it's not. Apparently, many of us have developed a strong spiritual side over the years. Many of these spirited women I spoke to are comfortable breaking out of the mold of conventional thinking and offered the following observations:

- "My children waited on top of the mountain. My boy came down first; my girl will be next."
- "One day I was lying by the sea, and all of a sudden, I had the very real and strong feeling that there was a baby around me, a spirit baby. This was not a hallucination; it was a very real feeling."
- "My mother and my sister have come back to me in my twins."
- "I was in the living room with my two children when I heard another baby cry upstairs. I literally heard Melissa months before she was conceived."
- "When we looked around the table, it was like one person was missing."
- "I hear the voice of God telling me that we have a second child coming to us."
- "'She is beautiful beyond words, and we are happy that she chose us to watch her grow over the coming years."
- "I dreamt of looking at a photograph of myself, my husband, our 4-year-old daughter, and a boy who was about 2 years old. We were all dressed up and smiling, and I thought, 'How strange,' as we only had our little daughter by then. A little later, I found out I was pregnant."

All these quotes come from accomplished women who have their feet firmly on the ground. One runs a five-star resort in Jackson Hole, Wyoming; others are an accomplished journalist, a children's rights lawyer, a successful entrepreneur, a real estate agent, an academic, an ER nurse, and a TV personality. Their statements are reflections of their worldview—that there is a soul-to-soul connection between parents and their future children and that babies (their soul, their spirit) potentially have a say in whom their parents will be—and it also shows that these women are deeply rooted in one of our strongest feminine powers: the power to receive, whether it be messages, creative ideas, or children.

After mindfully making space in their own lives for creating life and welcoming a baby, many of the women I spoke to instinctively allowed their own intuition to come forth. They started to listen to their inner voice and inner guidance and started to receive information about their children in their dreams, through certain feelings that arose, or through events and meetings with other people who had special meaning, though it may have seemed random at the time. What seemed like a tiny spark inside them at first often grew into a strong sense of knowing that the spirit of a child who wanted to be born was close. If you, too, receive dreams of your child or feel a "presence" close by, believe us: you are not hallucinating—and you are not alone.

For Monique, the voice in her head was the voice of God telling her that they had a second child coming. For Rebecca, it was also God she felt coming through and who connected her with her child. Shule had a full-blown vision of her daughter, Sufia, while traversing the Arizona desert.

As you read in chapter 13, Claudia Spahr started reading the book *Spirit Babies* when she first felt the presence of her oldest son. She drew comfort in how the author, the late Walter Makichen, explains why miscarriages occur and what they can signify. (Claudia had lost her very first pregnancy.) And she stopped putting a timer on her conception once she realized that there is no sense of time on the other side. Not that much longer, Claudia fell pregnant again and, in her 40s, successfully carried all her subsequent children to term.

Another woman who drew great strength from the book *Spirit Babies* was Nancy Mae, who is now the author of *The Energetic Fertility Method* and creator of an online course of the same name. Nancy, herself, worked with Walter Makichen after she was diagnosed with unexplained secondary infertility (the inability to get pregnant a second time). She eventually conceived a baby spirit Walter had seen in their sessions. Nancy became one of Walter's trusted students, and she now connects future parents with their spirit babies.

After reading *Spirit Babies* myself, I was very curious about the communication with our future children (is this really possible?), and I reached out to Nancy, a former researcher at Microsoft who went from working with data to working with energy, to schedule a session. According to Nancy and other fertility coaches who focus on the more spiritual aspect of conception, we can "call a baby spirit in" if this baby spirit feels comfortable with us. My conversation with Nancy was *very* interesting, to say the least. If the topic of communicating with your unborn or even preconceived child interests you, please listen to my interview with Nancy in the resource membership area at *BettinaGordon.com/Bonus.*

Listen Closely, *Very* Closely

All the women in my book have gone on to become mothers, which does not mean that all the women I spoke to recognized that motherhood was, indeed, the right path for them. You, yourself, may think that motherhood is what you really want, yet once you follow the steps—finding your "I am going to be okay," surrendering to a process you cannot control, and starting to listen to your inner guidance—you may recognize kernels of doubt as to whether this is what you really want. It's a great blessing if you are able to realize your heart's true desire before it's too late.

I've spoken to plenty of women who started to listen to their intuition and their inner guidance and realized that starting a family might not be what they desired after all. One prime example is Divine Living founder and success coach Gina DeVee, who thought all through her 20s and 30s that she would be a mother one day. So, once she turned 40, she declared to her husband that, "This is it. It's time." Gina and her husband started getting ready when, one night, Gina went to dinner in New York City with a very wise friend named Regena Thomashauer, otherwise known as Mama Gena of the School of Womanly Arts.

Gina spoke about wanting to have kids, and seasoned Regena looked at her and said, "Unless you must—don't." Gina took this advice to heart and went on a deep soul search. Eventually, she decided to forgo her previous desire for having kids to live the life she is leading today.

My spiritual mentor, former New York City schoolteacher and owner of the metaphysical store Planet Earth, Lorraine Simone, had two miscarriages when married to her then husband in her 20s. At age 42, Lorraine met the man who she thought would become the father of her child. Then, something serendipitous happened, and her life went in a very different direction. Lorraine had the spiritual wherewithal to recognize what was happening, and she followed her inner guidance to create a spiritual community on the East End of Long Island. Almost three decades later, Lorraine has mothered hundreds of women and men and has created a loving and thriving community called Moonfire Meeting House and the Mystery School of Women's Ways in Southampton, New York.

"Could you have done this if you'd been a mother to one or two biological children?" I asked her recently. She shook her head and said, "You know, my path really turned out to be what I recognized it to be early on in my life but didn't have the vocabulary and didn't have the modeling or the support for it. My path is really to be the universal mother of all children." You can read more about Gina and Lorraine in my companion guide for this book, *Sisterhood*, which you will also find in your book bonus section on my website.

We all receive unique guidance and hear different messages once we tune into the divine. Whether you decide to become a mother one day or choose to take a different path, remember a poem by Guillaume Apollinaire. A male voice asks a group of people to come to the edge of what seems like a very steep cliff. But they are frightened and won't take the step forward. He encourages them again, and still they are too afraid to come closer in case they might fall. One last time he asks them to step to the edge. And they finally do:

And he pushed them.
And they flew.

CHAPTER 16

Claudia C.

One of the biggest lessons I learned when speaking to dozens of women was this: there is always, and I mean *always*, a story behind the 30+ or 40+ woman we see walking down the street, hugging her baby close to her chest. There is always a story to the mature mother pushing her toddler on the playground swing and the accomplished-looking woman who gently tugs her little one out of the stroller. We often tend to think that pregnancy happens in a snap, but that's not true. For most of us, it is a process, a progression, a marathon rather than a sprint.

I am grateful to Claudia Chan for sharing her story here. It would be easy to look at her and simply see the successful entrepreneur and women's empowerment and gender equality activist that she is, someone who topped off her career and life with a baby boy at age 40. Just a couple of months ago, Claudia stood on stage at the mega-event she produces once a year—the S.H.E. Summit in New York City—and rocked her second baby bump in a jade green dress with matching high heels and a megawatt smile for twelve hours a day. She was 41. When this book is published, Claudia will be mom to two children and will undoubtedly have become an even bigger power player in her world, empowering female and male leaders worldwide to rise to their highest potential while lifting up others in the process. Picture perfect, right?

Truth is, only two years ago, Claudia stood on the very same stage, opening her biggest professional event of the year, struck with the sinking feeling that she was about to miscarry her very first pregnancy—right at that moment. Nevertheless, she executed the whole first day of the event before crawling into bed with excruciating belly pain.

Against the advice of her doctor, she continued to moderate multiple panel discussions on the second day before finally checking herself into the hospital. "I remember being in the ER office at the hospital and staring at the ultrasound screen," Claudia recalls, "but there was nothing there anymore. I was so sad, and I was so sad for John, my husband, who was with me. You know, it's the woman's responsibility to carry the baby to term. It's my body, it's my energy, it's my life force carrying this child, so I was feeling that I had also taken something away from him. That's what it felt like. It was definitely one of the hardest experiences of my life."

Bettina: Thank you for being so candid with your experience. Can you walk us back a bit on how the whole journey to motherhood started for you?

Sure. I met John when I was in my early- to mid-30s, but we did not get married until I was 37 and he was 39. We were so passionate about our careers and focused on our own stuff that we took our time, and even after our wedding, I pushed the whole baby-making thing off for another two years. Then something surprising happened: we had spent so many years avoiding getting pregnant, and yet we expected to get pregnant immediately. That's not what happened, and after a couple of periods, I actively started looking for people to help me optimize my body for pregnancy.

I am very much a woman who wants to collect information and data so I can quickly make a decision and execute. That's when I found Aimee Raupp's clinic in Manhattan. I remember Aimee asking me all these questions about my lifestyle and what I was eating, my digestion, my habits, etc. Working with Aimee also made me realize that, before pregnancy was even possible, I needed to seriously slow down and get on the same page with my partner—and that I needed to have patience, as the process can take a while.

I think that's an important message. We are in a very powerful time for women—we are so extraordinary in what we are getting done. There is a major woman's movement, and it's all about "lean in" and be a "girl boss" and "change the world." We are working harder than ever, and we have more on us. It's not easy to all of a sudden pause and shift into this "other new thing" of starting a family. It even takes time for you and your partner to get on the same page. And even when you are on the same page, it's still all on us women. We are the ones who are tracking our temperature, our ovulation, etc.

Your own personal slowing down and shifting into this other state, calming down after going one-hundred miles an hour and becoming less stressed and getting in harmony with your partner—it all takes time, and we women need to acknowledge this. Getting pregnant may take months or even a year or longer, and we need to be okay with that and see it as a process, not a singular event. I am also the kind of person who has always exercised some control over her life. You can control your career to a large extent or what you manifest in your life to a certain degree. But when it comes to pregnancy and birth and breastfeeding, you realize that this is just not something you can control! And women are planners, and women like to have control. It's our comfort zone. But it does not work when it comes to anything baby related. So, I think the word "surrender" is the most powerful and appropriate word to use in this process. Surrender.

How long did it take for you to fall pregnant the first time?

Well, I had Aimee by then, and she helped me to chill out and not get too stressed in the process. She taught me that I was not alone. We see other pregnant women and often assume that it just happened quickly. But that's not true. For most of us, it is a process, not an instantaneous event. We need a kind of chill attitude and the recognition that this will take time, and we need to be okay with that—going with the flow, instead of getting more and more stressed, which will prevent you from getting pregnant when your body is all flooded with stress hormones, right? So much about pregnancy is in the mind and in the emotions and, of course, the physical body.

I fell pregnant within a few months of working with Aimee. When we found out, we were in this really insane few months before the S.H.E. Summit, which was happening in June of that year. The summit is a massive undertaking—it's like my Oscars. Our business, our company, our revenues, it's all tied in with this big event. The few months prior, my team and I were just hustling to get this huge conference produced. That's when my husband and I found out we were pregnant. But we were so paranoid, we did not tell anybody, not even my mom.

On the first day of the event, just before my big welcome speech, I went to the bathroom, and I saw blood. And I knew that this was not a good sign, of course. Yet I had to go on stage, and I actually executed the whole first day of the conference. I was bleeding throughout—it did not stop. I had excruciating belly pains, and I remember texting with and talking to Aimee that evening. The next day, my OB/GYN wanted me to go to the hospital, but being the crazy person that I am, I still went to the conference and moderated a few panels before checking myself into the ER at midday.

Miscarrying was hard, of course, and the timing was just so wild. It happened right at the beginning of the summit, not on the second day, not right after. So immediately, I went into thinking: Had I been working too hard? Had I been pushing too much? Did I cause this? Did I do this to myself? I was wondering if I had pushed myself so hard that my body could not hold the pregnancy. It was shocking. It was surreal. There were a lot of subconscious feelings, and then we were just so sad. It was definitely one of the hardest experiences of my life.

How did you recover from it?

Here's the thing about me: I am very spiritual. I am rooted in Christianity and in God. It was really hard when it was happening and the few days after, but the timing of it was just so uncanny. Because I'm so spiritual, I realized that I was meant to go through this experience. Like all other difficult experiences in my life, I believe I underwent it in order to understand the pain and suffering that so many other women go through so that I could expand my resources and support others. This is why I've had fertility and maternity as topics of conversation at the subsequent S.H.E. Summits. Miscarriages happen so very often, and we need to remove the taboo around it and talk about it openly, like I am doing now. Miscarriage is horrible, but it's common.

Looking back, the miscarriage is such a part of who I am. I am grateful for my biggest challenges in life, because our struggles and hardships and adversities are what build us and cultivate us and what, in turn, form our character. They give us the endurance we need to really do extraordinary things—and we are born to be extraordinary. It's supposed to be hard, and there will be work involved, and that's when surrender comes in. You begin to change your relationship to the hard things that happen.

Your spirituality was the foundation for your healing?

Yes. We cannot understand everything that's going on in our lives from our human perspective. There is a greater spiritual force out there that we cannot explain, so I believe it's better to surrender than to fight what is happening. If you don't have a spiritual belief, if you don't have that self-love and that surrender when something like a miscarriage happens, then you will continue to beat yourself up and hurt yourself. And that's not good for anything. It's not good if you try to conceive again; it's not good for your relationship with your spouse; it's not good for your career; and it's not good for your confidence, your identity, your self-worth.

It's easy to get caught up in the rat race. And what we think affects how we feel, and how we feel affects how we behave. Our thoughts are so powerful that we have to be strategic about what we let in. And our tendency as human beings is to be negative and to react to obstacles in a fearful way—to not feel that we actually have what it takes. So, having a practice, whatever it is, that shifts you back into your optimal mental, physical, and emotional state is absolutely critical. If you are rooted in something bigger than yourself, what you can achieve and all you are able to surrender is truly extraordinary.

On a more "earthly" level, I recommend going on vacation after an experience like a miscarriage. We went to Argentina. A miscarriage disconnects you, so you need to find your way back into the relationship, to drink wine and enjoy yourself. Within two or three months after losing the first pregnancy, I was pregnant again.

Oh, one more thought. It's so funny how we think, "Oh, the pregnancy and then the birth and having the baby, and then it's finally done!" But then you realize, no, it's just the beginning! Raising a child is no small feat.

Have you felt any negative judgment around pregnancy in your 40s?

Not at all, in fact, it's the opposite for me. I am proud to be a 40+ mom. I have never been one to worry too much about my biological clock. I feel like I am a late bloomer in everything, and I am so happy and proud to have conceived when I was 40 the first time and at 41 the second. I feel we need to see the women who design their lives differently than most and hear their stories. It's important to have role models for all these different opportunities, like having children later in life and also living longer.

I was six months pregnant at the last S.H.E. Summit, and I proudly wore my high heels and my belly on stage for twelve hours a day. Because I am so rooted in a foundation of spirituality and knowing who I am and what my values are, I was able to invest my time in what matters most to me besides my unborn child and my infant son. So, I still birthed this big conference while having a baby, and I proudly stood on stage to show the women that this is possible and that you don't have to freak out at 30-something when you are not even close to having a child. You have time.

What else did you learn on your journey to motherhood?

Honoring your body and your health helps you age in a way that preserves your fertility. Regardless of your age, the most important thing to do *before* pregnancy is to get into the best physical, emotional, and psychological state and to make sure you are really healthy in the mind, the heart, and the body. The more you focus on something, the more you get out of it. If you focus on fear and punishing yourself, the more you put that into your reality.

So be very conscious and strategic with the company you keep. Surround yourself with people who believe in you and who are positive. Be mindful with the things that you read up on and look for information that is supportive and won't get you down. Be very attentive and minimize anything that's toxic in your life, like people and energies. I know women who finally got pregnant after leaving their jobs because they were in really toxic work environments! And, ideally, don't do it alone. Seek out other women who are in similar situations. Aimee taught me that women in support groups get pregnant twice as fast as those who are not. Choose your company wisely.

And last but not least, don't leave the workforce. Having a baby means you will pay a lot of money for a doula, a midwife, a wet nurse, a nanny, an au pair, and whomever you choose to support you. It's expensive, but this support system is incredibly important so you can go out there into the world and still do what you do with passion and force and drive. You are investing in yourself as the vessel that holds it all together, as a mother, a wife, a daughter/sister/friend, and a person who brings her gift to the world. So, you can still go out there and be who you have always been, feeding your vocation, doing what you do for a living, pursuing your dreams, power, and purpose. I have it all—a child and a career that I am more passionate about than anything—because I surround myself with the very best support system I can get and because I invest in resources. Invest in the right people to support you.

CHAPTER 17

Stella

Not every woman I was eager to interview for this book was as eager to be interviewed. Stella is one of the ladies I had to be especially persistent with because reading her story in print was not high on her list of priorities. Her cousin, who had made the connection, already warned me that Stella, by nature, was a private person. But I persisted, and I am so happy I did, as this woman's story speaks deeply to the power and potential of having faith in God. And of taking matters—or, in this case, the Bible—into your own hands and transmuting scripture into your personal benevolent guide, something that speaks to you and to you only.

Stella is an African American woman with a strong, clear voice and a level head on her shoulders. She was born in 1970, the same year I was born five-thousand miles away across the Atlantic. Stella grew up in Maryland before moving north and settling down outside of New York City, where she has lived for the last twenty years. She has a high-level executive job in the world of advertising and marketing, and with the arrival of her daughter, Hope, only two months before her 44th birthday, her plate is more than full. But, then again, not full enough to not consider trying for Baby Number Two sometime soon.

Stella: I kind of always assumed I would be married and have kids, although my parents never pressured me about it. I was not stressed about it and happily embarked on my career in my late 20s. I got caught up with work and living my life, and it was not until my mid-30s that I thought, "Hey, wait a minute; I need to think more deliberately about my life if I want to marry and have a family."

When I met Michael at a big New Year's Eve party, we started dating, even though he lived on the West Coast and his work for the military had him traveling a fair amount. After four years of dating, he was moved to Boston, which was great. We got engaged, and we were planning on having a big wedding, but then we married quickly because there was a chance he would be deployed to Afghanistan, which thankfully never happened. But for the first two years of our marriage, he lived in Boston while I was in New York. It was not until his retirement that we moved in together. Until then, we did not actively try to get pregnant.

Bettina: That's interesting because, by then, you were well into your 40s. Does that mean you never heard a biological clock tick?

No, I didn't. That's not to say I was not thinking about getting older, but I wasn't stressed out about it. I am a person of faith, and I strongly believe that my life is in God's hands. And I believed that it was God's will that I have a child. So, I looked at certain scriptures in the Bible on the topic of marriage and family, and I internalized them. I was so sure in my belief that I did not waiver, and no doubt entered my mind. So, I cannot even speculate as to what would have happened if it hadn't happened. The pregnancy, I mean.

One of my favorite scripture verses says, "Faith is the evidence of things not seen." In other words, if it's one of God's promises, you can stand on that promise, and you can call into being that which does not exist yet and treat it like it is real and true. You are convinced that it is real, even though it has not yet manifested. And so, that was my mindset. There was and is no space for "what if it does not happen?"

Outstanding. So, your faith in God's plan for you to have a healthy child was what kept you from getting stressed out?

Correct. I did not waiver in this mindset, not even when we lost the first pregnancy. But allow me to back up a little. Michael moved in with me in September. My days were full with work and running a household, but I also wanted to take a Bible college course twice a week in the evenings. That was important to me, as I grew up in a family of faith. We went to church together, and I've been an on-again, off-again student of the Bible all my life, not from a doctoral perspective but from the understanding of and having a relationship with God and Jesus. The timing was a bit stressful, as Michael and I had just found our footing together as a couple under one roof, and I already had a demanding job and a long commute home, and the course made my evenings even longer. Despite all of this, Michael agreed it would be good for me to pursue my passion to learn more about the Bible.

I strongly felt that this study was going to bear fruit in my life, and in the back of my mind, I felt that maybe the fruit it might bear would not just be in my walk with the Lord but maybe also a child. I surrounded myself with like-minded people who shared my faith, and we were learning together. I actually had intended to also prepare for pregnancy physically, like working out and cooking healthy foods, but I was so exhausted every night that I actually never did. Prayer was the only preparation I did. The study group was a wonderful experience, and lo and behold, I became pregnant right away. We were elated and grateful to have been blessed. Unfortunately, we lost the baby about six to seven weeks into the pregnancy.

Did that trouble your relationship with God? The sister of a dear friend of mine is also a strong believer in God, and she totally fell apart after her miscarriage. She now blames God for taking her child away and believes that God does not want her to have a second child. She is very angry.

I am very sorry to hear that. For me, no, this experience did not influence me in a negative way. It was hard and obviously tragic, but my faith was so deep that I did not fall into despair. I still felt that I would be okay, that we would be okay. Pregnancy for me has two dimensions: the physical and the spiritual. On a physical level, I felt encouraged because my OB/GYN was impressed by how quickly I had gotten pregnant, and she was not worried about the miscarriage, as miscarriages are fairly common. She was not concerned—she just said to wait a couple of months to try again.

From the perspective of faith, and this is really where my head lies, I was thinking, "I so strongly believe God wants me to have a baby—so what can I be doing to help the process?" This is when I went from reading the Bible to really, truly digging deep and making certain scriptures my own. I searched for the scriptures that talked about motherhood and God blessing the womb and that there would be no miscarriages. I stood on certain scriptures and made them my own. They were written for *me*.

For example, in Psalm 91, there are words of protection that read like, "That no evil will befall you, that no pestilence will overtake you, a thousand may fall by your right, then thousands on your left, but it will not overtake you. Goodness and mercy shall follow you all the days of your life and you will dwell in the house of the Lord forever." Verses like that I pulled out of the Bible and read them out loud before and after I conceived my daughter.

Before the miscarriage, I was reading the Bible, but I had not made the scriptures mine, and this time I did. They were *my* scriptures; they were written for *me*, and I was serious about them and read them all the time. Did I believe it out of necessity? Maybe, but whatever the reason, this is what I believed, and this is what made the difference for me. I did not lose faith; I deepened it. Three months after the miscarriage, I was pregnant again.

How was the pregnancy?

Wonderful. Because of the experience of the miscarriage, I waited until week eleven to go and see the doctor for the first time. When we did the sonogram, we had the same technician, and she remembered me. She had the monitor facing her at first, and as soon as she saw that the baby was healthy, she whipped the monitor around and blurted out, "That's a healthy baby!" so that I would not be in suspense any longer—so sweet. I'll never forget the image, because Hope's little hands and legs were moving, and she's a mover still to this day.

My pregnancy was really good. My stomach felt uneasy at times, but I never had to throw up. I was averse to certain smells and became a fanatic about cranberry juice. Funnily enough, I lost my sweet tooth as foods became too sweet for me, and so I did not gain much until the very end, when I gained more in the last month than I had previously. Hope was born a couple of months before I turned 44.

Was your age a concern for your medical team, and if so, how did you deal with that?

I never doubted my body's ability to conceive and carry a child, but I exercised the caution I learned through my faith when I was dealing with my doctor and the specialists I was sent to because of my age. I was careful not to internalize things that they said that could have left me worried or anxious, thinking about all the what ifs that weren›t good. It's funny, but you have to be very careful about what you feed your mind, because even the most well-meaning people will say things to you that can degrade your faith. I think you have to become even more protective if you are a mom–to-be over 35. It's not that the medical professionals are all cynical—they have to tell you all the risks based on the odds, and they do. But, as the recipient of these negative messages, we have to be very careful not to let them into our minds and bodies. Otherwise, it will degrade our faith in the love, mercy, and power of God through his Son, Jesus Christ.

You really have to make a decision here: are you a woman of faith or not? If you are, then you need to be very discerning and not let in the negativity that can crumble it. That's also true for well-meaning people who love you, as they can also say things that will have a negative impact on you. Maybe even more so, because you know they come from a place of love and you trust them. So, I often and routinely change the subject if a conversation touches on a topic that I need to protect, like my faith or my faith in God's plan for me to have children. Besides, we all most likely already know the information on later motherhood that's out there, but I chose not to think about that and not to give this information a place in my head or my heart or my body. This can sometimes cause you to censor things, but I had to do it to protect my faith and my pregnancy.

Give me an example, please.

Gladly. When I was getting closer to my delivery date, my doctor said that I should be induced before the full term of forty weeks was over because I was over 40. That surprised me because there was never a time that my medical team was concerned about anything during my pregnancy. I asked them if they saw something in the tests that concerned them. They said, no, but the statistics have shown . . . blah, blah. I said, "I hear you. I understand. But these are statistics and odds, and I want to know if you see anything personally in me or my results that gives you the feeling you need to intervene." The answer was, "No, but . . ." So, we went back and forth and negotiated. I agreed to be induced, but no earlier than forty weeks.

This is just an example of how people mean well—they were good doctors and were doing what they thought was best—but what was driving them was fear that was based on statistics and not based on me or my results. So, we agreed to forty weeks, and I was induced, and Hope was born the morning after her due date. All went well!

Congratulations again; that's great. Now, at 46, are you guys thinking of giving Hope a sibling?

Yes, absolutely. I'd like to start trying soon. But before that, we need to figure out the sleep thing as she still does not sleep through the night, and I cannot picture myself getting up for Hope and a second baby. I am much too tired for that. I need to let her cry it out, I know, but so far, I have not been able to do that. I am such a sucker. But I know I need to do this and move on. Hope is definitely a child who loves other children and hugs and kisses them. She needs a little brother or sister, and I believe that the same thing that happened last time will happen again—so that's where I am.

You just brought a huge smile to my face. Please be in touch and let us know when Hope is going to be an older sister!

CHAPTER 18

Tamara

Being from Europe myself, I made a conscious effort to find women who were born or were currently living outside of the United States, as I wanted to collect as many diverse perspectives as possible. When I dove into my interviews, one woman was right at the top of my wish list: German-born Tamara, whose photo I had seen on Facebook when a mutual friend connected us. Tamara was 38 and a half when her daughter was born and 40 and 43 when her sons followed. When I eventually met this fetching blue-eyed, red-haired lady via Skype, our conversation turned out to be inspiring, and I learned a lot about a mother's instinct and the courage to follow it against the mainstream.

Tamara met her future husband, Oliver, an American, while they were both starting a new life in Los Angeles. She was there as an exchange student and made money on the side with dog walking, while he was finishing up his law studies and studying for his bar exam. "I was committed to Oliver, but I also struggled with questions like, 'Do I really want to get married?' and, 'Do I really want to have children?' Getting married and starting a family with Oliver was not a given for me," Tamara told me.

Instead, she finished her PhD in Pastoral Psychology Counseling and started working. The years went by, and Tamara was still on the fence until one fateful night, when, as Tamara describes it, "A door opened up, and I had the choice to walk through it, or not. One night I had this dream. I saw a little girl on a swing that hung from the branch of an apple tree. I watched her swing back and forth with this big smile on her face, and somehow, I realized that this was my daughter with Oliver."

Tamara fell silent for a moment during our interview. Then she added, "I am not a very spiritual person. In fact, I am rather careful with things of that nature. Yet I've come to the conclusion that there is something mystical about children and their parents and that there is a connection between them before the babies are even conceived. I dreamt of each one of my children before I was pregnant, or at least before I knew that I was, and I am not one who usually remembers dreams. In fact, the last seven years, I remember only three dreams: those of my three children."

I've heard it before in other interviews, but Tamara really illustrated it beautifully: when we well-educated women (let's admit it, we are thinkers, analyzing everything!) allow our analytical mind to rest for a moment, then we can hear the voice inside that knows what's possible for us. The voice can speak to us in our dreams or when we sit by the ocean or walk down a busy sidewalk. When we hear it, we have a choice: do we follow that voice or not? If there is one thing I learned from these interviews it's this: when we let our hearts lead, we are always led toward growth and love. The purest form of our female inner voice manifests as a mother's instinct toward her child—and this voice can be rather fierce.

Tamara: By 2009, I had decided to say yes to my daughter, and so Oliver and I got married to show our commitment. We were excited about the new direction of our lives, and we conceived our first child very, very quickly during our honeymoon. Sadly, this baby was not here to stay. The first sign of things going wrong came the day after we got back from our trip. Out of the blue, I was fired after being at my job for four years. I was dumbfounded, and I didn't handle the stress very well. At eleven weeks, we had an appointment with my gynecologist. He could not detect a heartbeat, and I realized that our baby had died. I was shocked.

Even though Oliver saw the miscarriage as being part of nature, I could not see it as such. For quite some time, I blamed myself for losing the baby, and I was wondering, if I had done things differently—like dealing with the loss of my job differently—could I have kept the pregnancy? Was this an indication that I may be too old by now to have children? By then I was in my late 30s, and I wondered if I would ever be able to get pregnant again. By the way, the baby's due date was right around my birthday in October. Every year since that loss, I've thought about my first baby on its due date. I think that if you'd ask a mother about *all* her children's birthdays, she could tell you.

Even though we suffered this loss, we still felt that we were on the right path, so we tried again, and I became pregnant quickly, just a few months after the miscarriage. Unfortunately, I was a nervous wreck because I was afraid to lose this pregnancy as well. I kept on thinking about a friend of mine who lost three pregnancies before she birthed her only child. Intellectually, I knew, of course, that her experience was no indication of what would happen to me, but when I was in this vulnerable space, I could not help but wonder if I'd lose this baby too. Having been out of work did not help either, as I had no distraction from my worries.

In addition, I was very disappointed with my OB/GYN, whom I had initially liked a lot. But now that I was pregnant at age 38, he instilled a lot of fear in me, telling me, in detail, about all the risks and focusing on everything that could go wrong, instead of all the things that could go right. My advice to women who are conceiving after an age that is labeled "high risk": look for a medical team that is supportive and encouraging and dismiss anybody else who is not!

Bettina: You are absolutely right! Did you get a new OB/GYN as well?

Yes. I was so discouraged by my American doctor that I reached out to a female gynecologist in Germany, whom my family had known for many years. I found her advice to be solid, calm, and much more encouraging. I also asked friends of mine who had children about their experiences and how they ensured that the entry of their babies into this world was smooth and beautiful. I thought about the soul of my child and what I could do to help this being enter the world in the best way. Of course, that included where and how to deliver.

Remember how I said that I had lost my job right after our honeymoon? As a result, I did not have health insurance in Los Angeles, which was scary for me. A friend of mine, who also hadn't had insurance, needed three years to pay back the hospital bills from her delivery. So, Oliver and I decided that it would be better for our daughter to be born in Germany, where I still had insurance. Six weeks before Victoria arrived, I flew to Germany to be ready in time for her birth. I felt strong and healthy and had planned on a natural delivery. And, indeed, I delivered her with the help of a midwife, and it was a natural birth without any medication.

Victoria was still an infant when I felt intense pressure to have a second child. I think that pressure was age related, because we were nearing our 40s and were wondering what it would mean for our girl to have older parents. Admittedly, we also thought about a second child so that our firstborn would not be alone once we were gone. But there was also this dream I had again. It was a family portrait that I saw through the lens of the photographer. Oliver and I and our 4-year-old, Victoria, and a little boy, about 2 years old, was in the picture. I saw this in my dream. And guess what? A few years later we were all at a friends' wedding, and the photographer took the exact photo that I had dreamt about three years prior!

Did you conceive easily and quickly again?

Yes. We were all back in Los Angeles, and Victoria was such a delightful child—I could truly enjoy my second pregnancy. I was not stressed or nervous, nor did I have any other problems at all. So, I did not think of anything bad when we went to the nuchal translucency screening, which is a routine screening for all unborn babies. The test came back and showed possible birth defects. We were told that our son had Down syndrome or trisomy 13 or 18 or, in the best-case scenario, a heart or kidney defect. I remember crying and shaking and calling my sister to tell her. Our world shattered that day. As recommended by the doctor, we scheduled testing of the amniotic fluid, the amniocentesis.

Did you and Oliver know at that point what you would do if the baby had the life-threatening trisomy 13 or 18?

We were prepared to have a Down syndrome child and would happily have welcomed it. The trisomy 13 or 18 was much more difficult to come to terms with. We had friends who birthed their trisomy 13 child and watched it die a few days later, so we knew what a birth defect like that meant. We were really hoping we would never have to make a decision. And luckily, the results of the amniocentesis indicated that our baby would be born with either a heart or kidney defect, or both. I say "luckily" because the result could've been worse, but it was still an awful and very frightening diagnosis to hear. At that point, Oliver put his foot down and said, "No more tests; otherwise, we'll drive ourselves crazy!"

I had the diagnosis, but I was still praying that our child would be healthy and not have any birth defects at all. With great gratitude, I can say that Martin was born 100 percent healthy! He is rather big and muscular and strong, the true opposite of a weak child. But I've thought back on the diagnosis and our decision to do the amniocentesis many times since. And I concluded that doing the amniocentesis was a decision that I regret to this day. I had a bad feeling before the procedure, and I wish I would have listened to my instinct as a mother and not given in to the pressure of the doctor.

I believe that something happened to my child during the procedure. Martin was born healthy and is a lovely child, but he also cried for hours and hours on end for the first few months of his life. For two and a half years, he woke up eight to twelve times every single night, crying his heart out. It was gruesome! He also had trouble breathing, and there were many nights I would walk around with him in the fresh air outside so he could breathe. Martin is a child who reacts very strongly when anybody enters his space. It's like he has to defend himself, and he does it with all his might, using his hands and feet if necessary. He questions every rule he is given, and he defies it if it does not make sense to him. He lives his truth, and he lives it without fear. Martin will not bend.

My older son has many traits that are very demanding for me as his mother, but they will serve him well later in life. That's his personality. But there are traits, like his fierce need to defend himself, that I cannot help but connect to what happened during the amniocentesis. Can I prove it? No, but, as his mother, I have a very good understanding of who this child is, and I strongly feel that it was a mistake to go through with the testing. Something happened, and I would encourage every other woman to not go through with the needle testing if she feels she should not.

Did you do any testing during your third pregnancy?

No, we did not. Let me just back up for a moment. Right after Martin's birth, we decided that having two children was enough. We were done. I gave all the clothes and toys away as soon as Martin had outgrown them. We used the same contraceptive method we had used for almost fifteen years. We also decided as a family to move from Los Angeles to Germany, to Bavaria, to a little hamlet close to where I grew up. Due to Oliver's work schedule, the international move with our two young children fell squarely on my shoulders. Only a crazy person would decide, "Hey, this is a perfect time to have another kid," right? By then I was also 42. And yet, I had another dream *(laughing)*. I dreamt that I was in the kitchen in our house in Germany, preparing breakfast, and I saw myself putting three plates on the table for my children. "How strange," I thought. One week later, I found out I was pregnant. What timing!

Your story reminds me of the sentiments many other women shared with me, that our timing is often not the timing of the baby.

Right?! We were very surprised by the news but also embraced and loved our surprise right away. There was no doubt or hesitation, and frankly, there was also not much time for me to be worried or anxious about my third child's health. I had a transatlantic move to master, and I had to help my little ones acclimate to a new world basically all by myself. I did not have much time to worry. Oliver missed Leo's birth, unfortunately, but all went well, and it was my third natural birth at age 43.

Since you did not see yourself as a wife and mother for quite some time, let me ask you, was having children later in life a good decision for you?

This is a resounding *yes*! It was good for me because, by the time I had them, I wasn't afraid to miss out on anything. I had traveled, I had lived abroad, and I had met a variety of people all over the world. There is no urgency for my children to grow up so that my own life can start again. In fact, it is the opposite. I feel very relaxed with them, and I can give them all the time they need to grow. So being in my 40s is good for me, but it's also very beneficial for my children that I did not have them when I was in my 20s.

Back then, I was still so connected to the family system I had grown up in that I had never seen or experienced how other parents educate their children. That would have meant that I would not have had the courage to question my mother and father's parenting style, and I would have blindly demanded that my own children follow my rules as the authority figure. You see, my father was a pastor, and he demanded obedience. He was the one who heard the voice from God, and he gave us this voice. And our own voices, that of myself and my siblings, were systematically shut down.

But in the last fifteen years, I had a chance to learn from quite a few families through my work as a pastoral psychology counselor. I learned about their values, their systems, and their way of coping with challenges, and in turn, this knowledge made me confront my own past and my own upbringing. Today, I am choosing conscious parenting over authoritative parenting, and I challenge and scrutinize what I would have unquestionably accepted in my earlier years. I trust my mother's instinct, and I will speak up for what's right for my children—even if I offend others by doing so.

Your mother's instinct has quite a fierce voice, doesn't it?

Now, well into my 40s, I have the courage to challenge every authority, whether it be religious, medical, political, spiritual, or anyone in a position of power who tells us what we should do—something that I could not have done as a young woman. I scrutinize, and I don't follow blindly anymore. Let me give you an example. My pediatrician was promoting baby food enriched with iron, and he told me that this premade food was better for my children than my homemade food. Pardon me? Well, I started doing research, and I found out that my doctor has a lucrative contract with the producer of the baby food to promote their products. Years ago, I may have just gone with his suggestion and never doubted him. But as a mother, I feel much more of a responsibility to question authority than I would feel if I was only looking out for myself. Now, I question every level of authority. I am prepared to offend others and deal with the backlash, but I won't let my children down and go against what's true for us!

CHAPTER 19

Shule Marie

Religious texts are filled with stories of devout people who had visions and were visited by saints, prophets, and messengers who delivered news of great importance. If you are anything like me, you may have read about these encounters but never taken them too seriously. Well, that changed for me when I heard Shule's story. Just imagine: you are a 36-year-old woman, and you are driving—stone-cold sober and without the use of any vision-enhancing drugs, I might add—through the Arizona desert on your way to work in Los Angeles, when the figure of a young girl appears in front of you. Nonchalantly, she tells you that her name is Sufia and that she is your daughter. Excited and bewildered, you turn to your husband, who is behind the wheel, but before you have a chance to say anything, you suddenly realize that he is *not* the father of the child you literally see in front of you. You look at Sufia again as she delivers her loving and urgent message: "Okay, Mom, it's time to find Dad. I am ready to come— let's get this going."

Seriously, what would you do if that happened to you? Have faith or declare yourself nuts?

When my friend and coach Mindie Kniss connected me with Shule Marie Besher, I had already made up my mind to stretch my own criteria—only interviewing women who became moms in their 40s—by a couple of months.

Shule was just shy of her big 4-0 when she delivered the girl she had seen years before, and I wanted to know all about it. And because Mindie knew Shule, I could be reasonably assured that I would be speaking to a levelheaded woman with two feet on the ground—not some over-spiritual, pie-in-the-sky airhead who had made up her vision.

Here's the woman I found: Shule is a gutsy world traveler who first left home at age 17 to travel for seven consecutive years. A yogi, singer, and meditation teacher, she eventually became the CEO of a Canadian Health Center, and among other achievements, she led workshops with health guru Dr. Deepak Chopra. Shule has been striving to become the best and highest version of herself throughout her adult life, and she took care of herself physically, as well as mentally and emotionally, years before her daughter was even born.

After her vision in the Arizona desert, Shule took *a huge* leap of faith to find the man who was not only the ideal mate for her, but who would also be evolved and conscious enough to become father to little Sufia. Shule had to literally leave her old life in North America behind to make her vision come true, as her "beloved," her "destiny," was a man who was born half a world away. A Canadian beauty with long brown locks, with hints of gray, and hazel eyes, Shule now resides in Giza, Egypt's third largest city. Together with her second husband, Omar, she leads Activation Tours to the region's power-places, trips that are designed to elevate the consciousness of the group's participants. Shule and I were chatting on Skype when her daughter toddled over to join us, and yes, Sufia is turning into the spitting image of the girl Shule had seen while driving through the desert.

Bettina: Your story is pretty remarkable. Did you always think that someday you would be a mother, or did this vision come out of the blue?

At that point, I was not sure about having children. It had not been a strong yes or no for me, maybe because I had never had a man in my life with whom I wanted to have a child. Don't get me wrong. I loved my first husband, and we were married for seven years. We had a wonderful relationship that made us both grow in many ways, mainly because we brought out the dark side in each other. That was a massive gift, because I became a more authentic version of myself through our struggles and fights *(laughs)*.

I had gone off the pill years before when I realized how it messed with my hormones. My first husband and I talked about kids and did not use contraceptives. We had a very active sex life, but I never got pregnant. I know my body well, so I knew when I was ovulating, but every month, something would get in the way. We would fight, travel separately, or would otherwise be distracted during those times of fertility. I believe that we weren't energetically designed to procreate. Then, all of a sudden, during our drive through the desert, Sufia appeared in front of me. The experience was so intense, tears streamed down my face. When I looked at my partner, I knew in an instant that he was not the father. Thankfully, we are both very aware people, and we realized that our relationship had come to completion. Our separation ceremony was almost even more beautiful than our wedding.

Now there's a sentence I have never heard in my life.

And I am grateful for that as, from the moment I had seen this child, I thought, "Okay, there is a being who wants to be born through me. This is my responsibility now. I need to stay open to her and take very good care of myself and my body. And I will do whatever it takes to find her father and prepare for her arrival." So, I stayed open and let life guide me to Omar. Shortly after my vision, a woman contacted me and asked me to organize and co-lead a tour to Egypt—in four weeks, a crazy idea. But she knew this family that lived at the base of the famous pyramid of Giza, and they are pretty much the gatekeepers to Ancient Egypt. They had an opening, and so I said yes.

In the subsequent weeks, my wheels were spinning, and I was online constantly to make this happen. One day, Omar popped up on a chat and offered his help. The moment he appeared on my computer, I turned into a little girl. I was nervous, and there was such intense energy when we started speaking. I knew nothing of him and have no explanation for my reaction. He's just epic and beautiful, and I felt this very deep lifetime of connection with him. I told him about the changes that I sensed were coming and that a child was calling to me. I mean, I would talk to this man as openly as I talk to you now. And, of course, he knew it already. As he tells me, he'd been waiting for me. He saw I was still married, but that did not matter, as he knew all of this would be changing. So that was the beginning of our connection, three years before our daughter was born.

We met for the first time in person during this tour, and it was amazing. Sufia kept showing up for me in my dreams and meditations, and so I needed to have the baby conversation with Omar early on. I was in my late 30s, and she wanted to come—there was no time for a long courtship. In fact, we joke about how nothing about our courtship was typical. We basically went right into "we are going to have a baby," but he got it, and he felt it, and Sufia also began to show up in his dreams and his meditations. So, we trusted . . . but Omar is a little bit younger than me, so we also needed to wait for him to finish university and do a year of mandatory military service.

Hang on a second, university and military? How young is a little younger?

Fifteen years younger.

Cradle-robber!

Yes, we are laughing now, but we, indeed, had to overcome so many obstacles. There was the age gap, the fact that he grew up in an Islamic culture, the physical distance between Egypt and Canada—on paper, this just wasn't a good match. But we were so beyond these obstacles energetically and in how we related to one another that it allowed us to take a real leap of faith. I trusted that we would work through my worries.

I actually thought, at first, that it was totally inappropriate of me to basically steal this man's youth. That was the story that was going through my mind, that it would somehow be wrong or bad to do this. Thankfully, I had the maturity, the age, and the experience to work through my doubts. Omar has a spiritual depth to him, and culturally, Egypt is a place where you typically marry and have families very young. Young people rarely travel the world—most of them cannot even leave Egypt. So, his psychology at 22, the age he was when we first met, was much different than that of an American or Canadian man his age. He wanted a partner already, so that worked to our advantage.

When Omar and I came together, it was just so instantaneous. From the very beginning, we were making love to create life! We never did anything to block or to protect. I had never had this intention before with a man, but with Omar, regardless of whether I was ovulating or not, we were making love to create life, and it was just so beautiful—oh, so beautiful.

Years passed before you would conceive. Did you ever doubt that your pregnancy could happen?

No. When Omar was in my life, I never doubted. It was just a question of when. As you said, we actually had years together, but we were mostly separate because of his education and the military. Sufia came to me again just before I was going to go back to Egypt to lead a tour and be with Omar when he completed his year in the military. I was at a friend's house in Canada, and we meditated, and I came out of the meditation telling my friend when and where Sufia would be conceived. I told her the date, and I told her the location, and we laughed because she had been there. The location was the temple of the goddess Isis in Egypt. We laughed because, how were we going to do this? There are no corners you can sneak away to make love in, especially in an Islamic country. There was just no way.

The next day, I received a call from the other leader of the tour. "Shule, I found the most amazing camp with glamorous canvas tents and torch lights on a beautiful island just across from Isis's temple. Do you want to stay there?" The place was right in the vortex, the power-place, of Isis. The two nights we would be staying there coincided with my ovulation. It was all there. Crazy, huh?

On this tour, we had women from the Hummingbirth Ranch in Colorado who were working with their clients on conscious conception. They knew about Sufia and our intention, and we had about fifty people pray for us the night she was conceived in the tent across from Isis's temple. And I knew it instantly when it happened. Omar and I, we both knew. I could feel this heat running through my body, and sure enough, that was it. Even when the doctors tried to tell me my due date, because they think no woman actually knows when she conceives, I knew better. I had it already calculated, and she was actually born on that exact date, not when the doctors thought.

By then you were 39 years old and were considered a high-risk pregnancy.

Yes, and I told my doctors right from the get-go that I understood their need to tell me all the things connected to a high-risk pregnancy, but I didn't consider my pregnancy as such. Nor would I go through this pregnancy with such a mentality or think about the birth being high risk. My team was awesome, and the doctors went right with me and my attitude. They told me about available tests but did not push them.

It's interesting, though. Once you know you're going to have a baby, regardless of your age, there is really nothing you can do unless you would be willing to abort the pregnancy. Otherwise, you are going to have the baby, and the baby will be what it will be and will have whatever it's going to have. So, you either spend your pregnancy stressed out and worried about what may or may not happen at birth, or you just surrender to the process and trust that whatever is coming through you is coming through you.

That doesn't necessarily mean that everything is going to be fine—there are babies born with all kinds of issues—but there is really nothing you can do. And if you worry all the time, the body becomes nervous and contracts and stresses. The uterus also contracts, restricting blood flow and oxygen, and how does that affect the baby in utero? The baby gets less nutrients and oxygen, and what does that mean for the baby's brain? What can happen there in terms of disease? Whereas a woman who is relaxed, who is confident, who has faith, who is trusting her body . . . the blood flows, the oxygen flows, and she is conscious about what she is eating and putting into her body. What would you prefer for your baby? At this point, I should maybe mention that I was in Canada for much of my pregnancy, where I had fresh air and access to healthy and nutritious food. I also birthed Sufia in Canada.

You are a gutsy woman who obviously marches to the beat of her own drum. What is your personal opinion on motherhood over 40?

You mean because I wasn't scared? On the superficial side of things, my grandmother had a baby at age 45. I have a cousin who had two children, one at 43 and one at 45. Psychologically, having these examples in my world have helped strengthen my faith. But more important, I believe that, as a society, we make collective agreements about certain things. There are unspoken beliefs that most of us buy into without ever questioning them. As a society, it's agreed that what we read, what we see around us, what we create together, is the result of an unconscious agreement we make as a collective. I believe that we collectively agreed that dying in our 80s is a good time to die. There is a collective agreement that menopause is going to be difficult and that childbirth is going to be excruciatingly painful and probably the worst and most beautiful thing we'll ever experience.

I think there is also a collective agreement that to be pregnant later in life is dangerous or hard, if not impossible. Most of us conform to these collective agreements without ever questioning them. But there are people who live outside the constructed beliefs that we've created, and they are doing things like having babies naturally without fear at much older ages than 40, just as you did, Bettina. I, myself, don't buy into this specific collective agreement either. I am stronger and healthier than I have ever been before. There is a certain maturity, a greater ability to commit to myself and my health and my wellbeing now at 40 than in previous decades. And I just recently read a study that kids born to older moms are stronger, healthier, and more educated, so why not focus on that fact for a change?

Are you, Omar, and Sufia ready for a second child?

I believe I will be shown when a second child is ready to come. Do we really believe it is actually up to us alone when we have children? I don't think we can superimpose a controlled reality onto a reality that cannot be controlled. If we are meant to give birth and to bring life to this world, we will, and it will happen in its own timing. I believe babies are part of that choice as well—it is as much up to them as it is up to us.

And so, I don't think that we get to set the time. I was shown years ago that a baby spirit wanted to come through me, and I showed up and said yes, I will be there. But I did not try to dictate my own terms. Through most of my adult life, I made choices based on my individual beliefs and experiences, rather than the collective agreements. And I am glad you are writing this book so that others have evidence that we don't all need to conform to the beliefs of the collective.

CHAPTER 20

Monique

Sometimes you see a woman and a word pops into your mind that instantly and often accurately describes her. For Monique, my word was "sassy." Tall, curvy, with her wild locks somewhat tamed into long braids that she throws into a messy bun, Monique does not just enter a room—she owns it. I had met Monique at my son's daycare and at neighborhood playgrounds and could make the African American beauty out from afar, usually by her chic and colorful clothes and her equally sassy and gorgeous 3-year-old daughter.

I had meant to ask her about her age in hopes she would fit my 40+ criteria but never found the right moment. It turned out I did not need to, as Jonathan, her fiancé—and unofficial spokesperson—started to talk to me at daycare one morning and happily and enthusiastically volunteered that their girl was the first child for both of them, that they were both in their 40s when they conceived, and that they were contemplating their second child. Oh, and that Monique had just turned 48 a couple of months ago. "But we were not the oldest couple when we attended our birthing class," Jonathan continued. "There was a pregnant lady who was in her early if not mid-50s there!" I smiled. Only a man can be so open about age, right?

Two days later, Monique and I sat down in my office in DC and talked about her experience, while Jonathan popped in and out of our conversation.

I've seen Monique with her daughter, so I could sense how much she enjoyed being a mom. By the same token, I was also not surprised to hear that she had initially made her career and travel her life's focus. "I did not want to have kids. I saw having children as being tied down," Monique explained. So, she lived independently and by herself for two decades before she met Jonathan.

They were pregnant within only two months of dating. Shortly after they found out, Jonathan moved in. Monique and her two Shih-Tzus were not quite sure how to handle the new person in their home and on their couch. "While Jonathan had cohabitated previously, I had never, ever lived with a man," Monique told me. "I would have been perfectly fine to continue our relationship between my house in DC and his house in Richmond, which is about one and a half hours away. But Jonathan is an all-or-nothing type of man, and so he moved in with me right after we found out I was pregnant."

"How did that go?" I asked.

"I needed to learn to share my house, my decisions, my accountability—basically everything—with somebody else."

"And?"

"Still learning."

Not only was it fun to speak to Monique and Jonathan, it was also interesting to hear how they managed to become and stay a committed couple after such a short courtship. And, once again, I got insight into the real story that was going on—the back-story, so to speak—when a woman says, "I was more focused on my career than on having children." In Monique's case, she had been a mother for almost her whole life, ever since she had taken over the parenting role for her younger sister while their own mom and dad worked all day. That's no small feat when you are 7 years old.

Monique: I grew up in a military family in New Jersey. Both my parents worked outside the home, so my little sister and I grew up as latchkey kids. When I was 7 and she was 3, I stepped into my role as her second mother. I learned to cook for her and not just one dish, but a protein, a starch, and vegetables for every meal. For example, I would make hamburgers and mac and cheese and mixed vegetables. I was there for my younger sister every day and took really good care of her. That was a lot of responsibility for a little kid like me, but somehow, I managed. In addition, I later on babysat the kids in our neighborhood. I was the busiest sophomore and junior in my high school, and I had the most money because I worked so much as a babysitter. Once I went off to college, that was it: no more kids, no more mother role. Looking back, I grew up more in adult mode than in kid mode, and I already had one child, my sister!

I dove into my work in telecommunications services, an industry that was really booming when I was in my 30s. I went from sales to product manager, and my career blossomed. I made very good money and established myself and my solid reputation here in the DC metropolitan area. I was very happy without kids. And, as a business coach I had been working with for a couple of years pointed out, I was not ready to have them. She said I should practice with a dog first. I dragged my feet for two years but eventually I bought my two Shih Tzus that I adore. They became the grandpuppies for my parents, and everybody loves them.

Bettina: What changed your mind?

Funnily enough, my sister. When we were young and played house, we both said that we would get married and have two girls each. Well, I did not want to hold up my end of the bargain at first, but she did get married before me. I was her maid of honor, and true to form, I took care of her on her special day as our mother needed to be with our grandmother. I helped with her dress, her makeup, her hair. I was the one handing her off, and I was more upset than my mother that day. I mourned that my baby was leaving. My sister had always relied on me for everything, from input into her clothes, to dating questions, to opening her bank account, and now here I was, handing her over to somebody else. I thought, "Wow, you now have a husband and not me anymore!"

I released her and grieved for my sister on her wedding day. And I looked at her in the years to come and saw how she designed a life with her husband that was different than what we'd seen as children with our parents. She created a different kind of marriage, one that was more appealing to me. They tried to have children but our grandmother got sick, and my sister helped out, and I believe that stress took a toll on her. I told her to relax, it's going to happen. The year after my grandmother passed, my sister got pregnant. And she was so beautiful in her pregnancy that I could not stop taking pictures of her.

When she gave birth, we were all initially there. She wanted a natural birth, but then she needed to be induced, and the medical team said that only one other person in the room was allowed. I immediately sprang into action, tried to control the room, and told them to dim the lights, put on some music, whatever. I did not even think once about my brother-in-law and that maybe he wanted to be there for the birth of his first child! I was totally ready, but my sister naturally chose her husband to be with her *(laughs)*.

I think my pivotal moment came right after she had birthed her beautiful daughter. Eventually we were all allowed to see them. I looked at my little sister, whom I thought of as my baby as well, and her little girl, and I saw her breastfeeding the child and doing all the natural things mothers do with their babies, and I thought, "Wow, I can do that too."

Did you have a suitable man in your life at that time?

No, so I started thinking about how I could do it. I considered artificial insemination, as a close gay friend had offered his help, so to speak. I thought I had some time to figure it out. My age was never a concern for me as all the women in my family are fertile. And even though they had their children earlier, I just did not think that I would have any trouble. I also believe that there is a spiritual aspect in having children. Children are a gift from God, a most beautiful gift that not everybody is blessed with. You really know it's God's work when you go to the doctor and see the sonogram and realize that what you see comes from an egg and sperm that all of a sudden turned into a human being. If people believe in the evolution side of mankind, everybody would be able to have children. But I think it's actually a gift to conceive and carry a baby. Of course, I did not know if I'd be gifted this gift as well, but my belief in God and that he wanted me to have a child was strong.

So, when I was 42 years old, I started to ask God to bless my womb. I was seeing a gentleman at that time who wanted to have children and having these conversations with him made it more real for me. We ended up breaking up, but it was probably his role in my life to really help me see myself in that way. He gave me the biggest compliment. He said that I had such a strong nurturing side and that I would be the best mom. I had never perceived myself in this way. When something comes so naturally and easily to you, you often cannot see it. He made me recognize it, which was wonderful.

So, I prayed to God to bless my womb so one day I would be blessed to have children. I prayed and affirmed: I am open and receptive to a loving and committed man who is emotionally available and has time to spend with me, a man who wants children, wants to be married, is spiritual, and family oriented. I prayed daily, and for two years, I asked God to bless my womb.

How beautiful.

In addition, I started to take really good care of myself physically. During a routine exam, my OB/GYN detected a fibroid in my uterus. So, I went to my naturopathic doctor who had known me for years. He said that fibroids love sugar and caffeine, so I watched what I ate. He wanted me to eliminate the coffee, get rid of the Mountain Dew and other sodas, watch the white sugar, lose about ten pounds, and detox the liver and other organs for twenty-one days. I also started to put a yam-based progesterone cream on my belly twice per day. Even if I did not meet the right person, my body needed to be healthy for my Plan B, the artificial insemination. So, I wanted to keep my body prepared for two years, as this just made sense to me.

Thankfully I did not read up on the internet about the negative stories concerning later pregnancies; otherwise, I would have only scared myself half to death. And I did not take to heart what my regular OB/GYN said. He was rather flippant and said things like, "You are not a spring chicken; we need to get moving," or, "You are up there; don't wait any longer," as if I could have pulled a father for my child out of thin air! I did my best not to listen, and I kept a very positive attitude and clean body for two years. The fibroid shrunk and was never a concern later on in getting pregnant. My pregnancy was a most wonderful experience as I had no issues at all, not even morning sickness, nothing. I was strong and healthy, and my child was born healthy and strong as well, only four days before my 45th birthday.

How did you and Jonathan meet, and how quickly were you pregnant?

We met through a matchmaking site on the internet. Jonathan asked me a lot of questions right away, which is unusual for a black man, as they are usually more evasive and get to these questions later. But on our first phone conversation, he already asked about my age—44 at the time, Jonathan is one year younger—and if I wanted to have children and start a family. And from our first date on, it was clear that this was it; we were a couple. It all happened very, very fast. We met in December, and I was pregnant in February. Jonathan, being an all-or-nothing type of man, gave up his place in Richmond and moved in with me. So, within a few very short months, my whole life got completely shaken up. All of a sudden, I was pregnant and had a man living with me. It was easier for Jonathan to become a couple and more challenging for me. I was used to being independent.

Jonathan: Overly independent!

Monique: And now I needed to share all the decision-making and how my life unfolded. I admit, I had a rather hard time with it and, on some level, still do. When Jonathan moved in, my perfectionism kicked in. I had this fairy-tale vision of getting married, having children, and of both partners having successful and thriving careers. I imagined jet-setting all over the world and having kids that were perfect and a life that was perfect. And any time my reality did not match up with the picture I had in my mind, I thought, "Oh, my gosh, this cannot be. I made a mistake!"

I also struggled with the fact that we had such a short courtship. Sure, before Skylar arrived we both said that we'd continue to go out and have fun, but all these good intentions quickly went out the window. I wanted Jonathan to date me again, to sweep me off my feet. Increasingly, I also had a hard time professionally, as I got bored. On the one hand, it was awesome that I was an independent realtor and could set my pace and bring baby Skylar with me when I showed houses, but I also missed the fast pace I had lived before and the social interactions I had when I still went into an office, which I no longer did.

So, I wanted Jonathan to read my mind and treat me like I wanted to be treated, and I did not want to feel like he was always telling me what to do. I wanted him to come up with what was wrong with me and fix it. I wanted him to think a certain way—*my* way.

You just eloquently described what many independent women feel in new relationships. With time, we all realize that relationships are never perfect and men are not mind readers.

So true. Sometimes when I get too frustrated, I think about being a single mom. But I don't want to be a statistic; I don't want to be yet another black single mom. In church, for example, there are really only two buckets you can fall into: you are either married or single. So, I prayed to God for guidance, and I talked to my mom and my sister who both attested, "Perfect does not exist!" Jonathan and I have had our hiccups in the last four years, but we've also grown. He challenges me to become a better person, something nobody else has really done before. And he, himself, is not afraid to change. When I saw him transform as a partner and father, I was able to change myself. I had to accept Jonathan for who he is and how he is and love him the way God loves him. Once I did that, everything else changed.

Obviously, there was also something divine about the way Jonathan and I had met and how quickly and easily we conceived. I had asked God for this man, and he brought him to me. So, be careful and prepared for what you ask for, because you may not know how quickly it is coming!

We are both committed to our daughter, Skylar, and that she should not grow up in a broken home. So, recently, we consciously recommitted to each other as a couple. We did a twenty-one-day fast, and we read scriptures and motivational literature together. The energy between us felt different, and we found solid ground. We are—and by that, I mean primarily me—finally ready to expand the *we* and get married in a small, intimate wedding this spring.

I also strongly feel that we will welcome another child. I actually hear it in my head, a voice telling me that we will. I hear God come through. I am going to turn 49 this year, and sometimes people ask me, "Why would you want to have a child so late?" or, "Are you not worried about genetic defects?" and I honestly don't understand these questions, because if we'd be given the gift of another child, it would be a blessing from God. Whatever is organically supposed to happen when a child is created is supposed to happen. A child is a gift from God that we would welcome and be truly grateful for. So, why wouldn't we want that?

CHAPTER 21

SPIRIT Action Steps

Choose Love and Peace over Fear and Drama

Becoming a spiritual person does not mean being the most enlightened, the calmest, the most collected, or the most compassionate woman in the room or the best meditator in town. The practice of being on a spiritual path is about surrendering to a higher power and connecting to a benevolent universe, a God, a divine power that only has our best interests at heart. I, personally, imagine there is a force field of divine love around us that we humans can connect to when we need it for strength and support. When we forget this force field of love exists, we feel lonely and fearful and quite literally disconnected from others, maybe even ourselves. Being on a spiritual quest means to choose this universal, unconditional love over the fear and drama in our minds, drama that we humans, sadly, are often addicted to. It means to choose love and peace over fright and crisis more often than the other way around.

If you believe that the miraculous creation of a baby is not just the result of your and your partner's bodily functions alone, then please look at this chapter as another item in your growing arsenal of tools that will help you conceive your desired baby, regardless of your age.

Being able to connect with a higher power and your own intuition and wisdom—and possibly your future children—requires all of us to become very aware of our lives and mindful of how we go about our daily tasks. It requires us to listen rather than speak, to receive rather than take action, to surrender rather than control. At first, most of us will have to slow down quite a bit in order to hear even a whisper. We may want to become more self-actualized and spiritual to enhance our chances of having a baby, but the benefits of all the action steps below will go far beyond fertility. Developing a practice of self-reflection, self-love, and mindfulness *now* will be immensely helpful once the little one has arrived and will benefit your child for the rest of her life. The actions on the following list may be your most important steps toward becoming the best version of a mother you can possibly be:

- A mother who makes her body and her physical and mental health a priority.
- A mother who treats herself with love and respect.
- A mother who is strong in her faith and who trusts her instincts and inner wisdom.
- A mother who is grounded and connected to the wisdom of nature.
- A mother who stands tall and speaks up for herself and her family.
- A mother strong enough to go against societal conventions if she feels she should.

Create Space for Your Future Child

If you Google "how to create space for your future child," you will get a myriad of tips on how to build an awesome nursery, even if you have the tiniest of apartments. That's not the "creating space" I mean. But I guess you've already figured that out.

When we mature women, who have a solid sense of who we are and what we can accomplish, desire to have children, something interesting often happens: we realize that the intensity and speed of our own lives has to change if we want to welcome another human being into our world. Intellectually, we realize this, but we try to rationalize: couldn't we make some room once the baby is here?

No, we can't. Again, you already know this deep inside.

If you are busy and occupied from dawn to late night, where is the space for a soul to join you? Seriously, if you feel that you cannot slow down now because you have so much on your plate, why would you think you'd be able to slow down for your baby later on? Or if you are financially stressed out right now, what makes you think you won't be like that once the baby is here? If you are burnt out by your job or your lifestyle, what can you give to a child?

Claudia Chang (chapter 16), founder of S.H.E. Summit, said it poignantly: "It takes time to personally slow down and shift into this other state, this state of creating new life. It takes time to calm down after going one-hundred miles an hour and to become less stressed and get in harmony with your partner. It all takes time, and we women need to acknowledge this. Getting pregnant may take months, a year, or even longer, and we need to be okay with that and see it as a process, not a singular event."

Slow down, my friend. Do it now, before you even get pregnant. Let's consider the many reasons why.

Just relax. *I am kidding.* Somewhat.

How often have you heard, "Just relax, and it will happen"? *Just relax?* Don't you want to slap the person who doles out such advice?

Urges of physical violence aside, you indeed need to step away from the one-hundred-miles-per-hour rat race so can you get in touch with your feelings and possibly connect to a higher power. This is not about blissing out in some Zen state; it's about allowing yourself to feel what is really going on—right here, right now. It is about catching yourself when you are frazzled and irritated so you can purposefully calm yourself down and relax. Let's take a quick excursion into our brain and autonomic nervous system to find out how.

One part of our brain is called the amygdala. The amygdala is the reptilian brain (the oldest, least sophisticated part) that goes into fight-or-flight response as soon as we are stressed. This stress can either be very real because we are threatened, like when a saber-toothed tiger chased our forefathers across the desert or our boss is about to fire us, or a perceived threat, like having the thoughts, "Nobody loves me," or, "My doctor told me I would have problems conceiving."

Unfortunately, your amygdala cannot distinguish between a real threat and an imagined threat and goes into fight-or-flight mode regardless. This means that your heart rate and blood pressure shoots up and that your body is pumped full of stress hormones like cortisol and epinephrine, drowning out your inner voice and grounded state. In our modern day, we have so many stressors (perceived and real), that our bodies stay in high alert almost constantly. And your body definitely won't let you get pregnant when there is a "tiger" on the loose!

Fortunately, there's an equal and opposite reaction to this fight-or-flight response called the relaxation response—also called the feed-and-breed (yes!) and the rest-and-digest response. In the relaxation response, all of those stress hormones go away, and the body releases healing hormones like oxytocin, dopamine, and endorphins. These are all hormones that help the body heal and to calm down—in other words, become less stressed. The body is beautifully equipped with natural self-repair mechanisms (which you need to boost your fertility, because it's an extension of health), and these mechanisms only operate when the body is in relaxation response. Any time your body's in stress response, those mechanisms are disabled. So, you want to learn and master how to turn on the relaxation response on purpose so that you can reap the benefits of a relaxed body and mind.

Breath. Meditate. Visualize.

One of the quickest and most effective ways of stimulating the body's relaxation response is by shifting your breathing rate and pattern. Even two minutes of mindful breathing will get you to a very different state than you were before. It can transform you from being frazzled and discombobulated to being strong and in charge of the situation. If you calm your breath, you can calm your mind and combat stress and anxiety.

Take a long, slow breath in through your nose, first filling your lower lungs and then your upper lungs. Hold your breath to the count of three. Exhale slowly through your mouth, while you relax the muscles in your face, jaw, shoulders, and stomach. Do this for two minutes, multiple times per day.

You may have heard about the benefits of meditation for years, just as I have. Meditation reduces stress and lowers blood pressure and heart rate. It increases self-awareness, happiness, and acceptance. It strengthens the immune system and cardiovascular health, and it slows down aging. Meditation is like medicine for your mind—it trains it to calm down and focus.

Sit or lie comfortably. Close your eyes. Make no effort to control your breath; simply breathe naturally. For beginners, it may be easier to focus on one single point, like following said breath, repeating a single word or mantra, staring at a candle flame, or counting the beads on a mala (string of beads). Find the meditation style that suits you best.

Visualization is another great way to stimulate the relaxation response and give yourself the chance to connect to your intuition and your inner wisdom, as opposed to searching for it outside of yourself. According to *Psychology Today*, anyone can utilize creative visualization to achieve a desired goal, like creating more work/life balance or attracting the ideal father for a child.

Turn your attention to an area in your life you want to focus on. After moving into deep relaxation, examine this area just as it is in your present reality. What do you most want to change about it? What emotions and feelings would you want to accompany this change? List all the reasons that prevent you from creating/having this reality. Is it fear, anxiety, too much disruption to your life or to your relationships? Keep on going until you have identified all of the limiting reasons. Now, imagine what you want to happen, unfolding as you want it to be. Set your desired goal. Listen to your inner guidance to affirm that what you are asking for is what you really want, is positive, and is meant for your highest good.

PS: You are actually a masterful meditator and visualizer already. You didn't know that? Then think about the many times you've visualized a situation going wrong or how you meditated (which is defined as having a thought over and over again) on a conflict from the past. We all focus, hence meditate, on negative stuff over and over again on a daily basis, without even being conscious of it. Well, not any longer!

Express Your Darker Thoughts

When you slow down and become real with yourself, many emotions and fears may bubble up to the surface. For example, if you've been on the path of trying to conceive for a while already, then let me ask you: Did you break out in tears when your close friend, coworker, or even your own sister announced her pregnancy? Were you ready to explode with anger because—again—it's not you who is pregnant and it's not fair that other women seem to have it so easy while you've been struggling for a long time now? If so, please know that what you are feeling has been felt by generations and generations of women before us. Feelings of jealousy, rage, victimhood, helplessness, envy, anger, not being understood, sadness, and loneliness and whatever other emotion a human being can experience have come up for countless women. The vast majority of them never talked about their thoughts and feelings because, well, it was culturally unacceptable to do so. That has to stop. Let's express these feelings and address them head-on, instead of keeping quiet and feeling lonely and isolated.

Hannah, mom at 42: "We did four in-uterine inseminations, but none of them worked. That's when I thought, 'Oh, great, I probably shot my chances; I can't have a baby anymore.' I was nearing 40 by then. It was about the same time my younger sister got easily pregnant and younger cousins and friends reported they were pregnant. That's when I started to feel more and more isolated from my friends and family. They were celebrating while I was feeling that I had possibly sabotaged myself. I hated them. I smiled at them and pretended to be happy, but I really only hated them. And I started to feel lonely, misunderstood, and hopeless."

Cara, mom at 40: "Not being able to have a child when you always anticipated having one is a *huge* disappointment. I was disappointed, but I also felt that I disappointed my parents and my spouse's parents and that, for the rest of my life, it would be awkward to see friends who had children. Suddenly, you go from someone who had an idea about herself to someone unable to bring a child into the community. That's awful."

This SPIRIT section is not about singing "Kumbaya" around the campfire or putting on a smiley face and pretending to be happy, while deep inside we are hurting, as Hannah, Cara, and so many other women clearly were. It's about acknowledging that our fighting spirits and our tender souls are often hurt in (literally) inconceivable ways on our paths to motherhood. It's healthy and vital to express our rage and our feelings and talk about them openly—just not, ideally, at the sister's baby shower.

Acknowledge and Heal What You've Been Through

Last winter I ran into an acquaintance of mine at the local supermarket. I knew that she was expecting, so while our two 3-year-olds ran off, we chatted. I noticed how slender she looked in her winter coat and said "Wow, you are carrying your pregnancy really well!"

And she looked at me and said, "I am actually not pregnant anymore. I lost the baby on New Year's Day, unfortunately—at eighteen weeks."

"Oh, my God, I am so sorry." And then I blurted out, "I had a miscarriage, too, on Christmas Day."

"Oh, how terrible. I am sorry," she said. As we looked at each other with deep sadness, I could not help but think that this was the most surreal conversation I had ever had in the middle of a busy supermarket. And that it was time we all began to speak about how losing a baby, however many weeks it lives inside our bodies, brings us pain and scares our spirit. How we deal with the hurt will determine if we get stuck in victimhood or take back our power of creation. Let's honor what we've been through so we can move on.

Let's stop pretending that we are fine if, instead, we are paralyzed by fear that we'll never have a baby or that we'll have more miscarriages or that this pain will never heal. Just now I read the posting of a mom who shared at #Ihadamisccarriage: "All I want to do is scream it to the world: *I had a miscarriage*, in hopes of feeling slightly less alone and a tiny bit less like a complete and utter failure at the only thing my body was biologically designed to be good at."

Let's allow ourselves to talk about our grief openly and fully. Let's talk about it even months or years later, even if people think, "Oh, it's six months already," or, "Hold on, you've given birth since." Regardless, if you need to talk about what you've lost a long time after it happened, do it. We need to be surrounded by people who will allow us to be very honest about our feelings, and we need to speak our truth openly and courageously. No more feeling alone and keeping numb.

As you know, many of the women who contributed to this book had their fair share of miscarriages and heartbreaks, and I am no exception. I had planned to surprise Joshua with a positive pregnancy test underneath the Christmas tree. Wouldn't that be the best gift he had ever gotten? Instead, I started bleeding the night before and was sullen, sad, and angry. Within a month's time, though, I realized that I did not want to hold on to these feelings any longer, as I had no time to waste if I wanted to give pregnancy another try.

Find Your Gifts

Slowing down and becoming more mindful may also mean that past wounds and hurts break open again. You may think you have dealt enough with the trauma in your life, but now is the time to look once again. Unresolved trauma can energetically get stuck in your body and, worse, manifest as sickness. These blockages influence your fertility and may block the unconditional love and tenderness you would otherwise have for your baby.

Please have the courage to look once more at how the experience of miscarriage, abortion, rape, or any other violation could still be "stuck" in your body, even though you thought you'd dealt with it (especially if you were diagnosed with unexplained infertility). Also, allow tears to flow. While it is possible to suppress grief and feelings of loss, it's not wise to do so. Release your tears now, before you carry your child in your body. A wise teacher once said, "Tears are the evidence that the soul is taking a shower." I've come to realize this to be true.

Once you've uncovered these blocks (most likely with professional help) and have identified the hurt, it's time for the next step. There are two parts to healing our wounds and, eventually, finding the positive in a situation:

1) First, the human part: It is very sad that the expectations we had for our pregnancy and the future with our child were not met. We created a picture that we wanted to step into, only to have this vision abruptly lost. Instead of keeping quiet and numbing ourselves with food, drugs, alcohol, sports, or whatever our particular vice might be, let's witness what we've been through and honor our grief and our anger and our sadness.

Break out your journal and write down all the emotions that come up for you on your journey. Dedicate your own "rage-rant" (or whatever you want to call it) journal, if you want. Writing it down will get the emotions from your head onto the paper and from your body out into the world. You need to say, "I am so disappointed, so sad about it," but in that disappointment and sadness, be careful not to give this loss undo significance. Avoid assigning it meaning like, "It's a tragedy"; "I am no good"; "This means it's never going to happen for me"; or, "This means I have failed and will permanently fail." Be very, very sad, because it is very sad. And be disappointed and angry and go deep into those healthy, affirming, self-protecting emotions, but do not take it to mean that the future is somehow tainted.

2) The second part to healing is the spiritual one. The pathway to healing occurs when you accept and love yourself so much that the darkness from the past can no longer dominate you. Honoring our pain and anger allows us to build a solid enough platform to then step onto the more spiritual level of it and look for the gift. We can question, how is this a gift? How can a miscarriage be a gift? How can being alone or not having found the right partner be a gift? What did this situation teach me? How did this open the door for me to become more than I was before?

For me, personally, the miscarriage made me realize, in no uncertain terms, that I need to take better care of my body and my health. Intellectually, I knew this (I mean, I wrote a substantial chunk of this book on exactly that), but now I also understood it physically. In my opinion, my miscarriage meant that Mother Nature had taken care of a fetus that was not of optimum health. I see the gift (I don't choose this world lightly) in the miscarriage as I would not want my child to be anything other than optimally healthy—and obviously there was a significant defect. I am not blaming myself, but I do take responsibility for my part. So, if I want to give my child the very best start into a healthy life, I need to considerably step up my health and self-care routine, which I have done ever since (more about that on my website).

After four years of trying to conceive, my friend Maria started to focus on the health of her relationship again. She and her husband had drifted apart, and she realized she wouldn't be able to give her child the upbringing she desired—a stable and loving two-parent home—if she kept focusing on getting pregnant and treating her husband as a sperm provider rather than a life partner. "I wanted to become a better wife in order to be a better mom," she said, and I never forgot that sentiment. Today, her daughter benefits from it.

Shortly after Rebecca gave birth to her son, her mother and sister passed within three months. Rebecca remembers, "When they passed, I was a brand-new mother for the first time who went through it all without her own mom, which was really hard. When I went back to work after a few months, I stopped making space for my grief for my mom and my sister and my process to heal." Two years later, Rebecca experienced the first of two miscarriages. "The miscarriage opened these wounds in a really intense way. It let me process my immense loss and my feelings years after my mother's passing, and I finally went through the stages of grief. Real healing came out of this experience, and so there was actually something positive about it all." At age 40, Rebecca welcomed naturally-conceived twin girls and named one of them after her beloved mother, Susan.

So, ask yourself: what was the gift in it? But don't start to look at it until you have fully grieved and allowed yourself to get really, really mad at the situation, because if you try to go the spiritual route before you do the human route, it will be false. It will be a way of suppressing your human side, and we don't want to do that because anything that's suppressed will stay and continue to contaminate our beautiful lives.

Connect to Mother Earth and Nature

We are born on the earth, and we will die on the earth. Nature and its bounty has sustained the developing human race for millions of years—it was only in the twentieth century that we drastically lost touch with nature's rhythms and teachings. But by now, in the twenty-first century, we can find plenty of scientific studies about the health benefits of being in nature—from boosting the immune system to improving focus and mood—and the benefits of, for example, gardening. (There are antidepressant microbes in the soil. Dirt literally makes us happy!). Personally, I think that the calming and grounding effect of nature is most beneficial for conception and pregnancy.

Go outside and walk in the fresh air for thirty minutes every day. Take in as much sun as possible during that time (which will boost your vitamin D level, which is essential for pregnancy). If you live in a large city, be especially vigilant to seek out nature daily and find your local parks and nature sanctuaries. Walk barefoot as often as you can and feel the grass beneath your feet. Squat down and touch some rocks and moss; let soil drop between your fingers. Lean your back on the trunk of a tree; close your eyes and wait for nature's wisdom to come your way. Let fresh air into your home and office as much as possible.

When you're on your daily nature walk, think of your baby and invite the baby into your life. Since there is often heaviness and pressure associated with creating a child, I suggest you make your outings especially lighthearted and fun. Chant or sing your baby into your life, skip down the path, throw pebbles in a pond, raise your head to the sun, stick your tongue out for snowflakes, jump into puddles in the rain, smile abundantly, and really, really enjoy your walks. Become a beacon that signals, "I am ready, and I am happy and fun to be with!" Make it light. I vividly remember when I jogged along the Danube river near my hometown in Austria a few years back, and I—with a huge smile on my face—asked the universe to send me a child that is bold and adventuresome and likes to travel. Guess I must have been a rather strong beacon that day. Every time my little adventurer, Hunter, runs off by himself now, exploring without any care of where his parents are, I wish I would have slightly adapted my request to the universe and added a "don't-run-off-alone" clause.

Once you have a child, you will see how often a crying baby calms down as soon as you go outside for a walk. We now have cutting-edge studies that conclude that direct exposure to nature is essential for a child's healthy physical and emotional development. On the other hand, the lack of nature in children's lives is linked to the rise in obesity, attention-deficit disorder, and depression. If you'd like to know more about the importance of outdoor time for children, I suggest the book *Last Child in the Woods* by Richard Louv.

Happiness Is a Choice

As a society, we are wired to seek happiness outside of ourselves. Happiness is the elusive state we may reach once our wishes are fulfilled, like once we get into the right university, land the dream job, connect with the ideal mate, have our baby, get the child into the right preschool . . . you get the picture. Happiness is something we chase and/or make dependent on our genes ("I was born a pessimist.") and our environment ("I cannot possibly feel happy; look at what's going on around me."). I, too, have fantasies about a second baby and how happy it would make me to finally hold the child I so long for in my arms. Are you tying your happiness to your future baby as well? Are you envisioning a future in which you'll be happy when a certain event has occurred or a dream is realized?

"We got it at all wrong," Shawn Achor, the famed expert on Positive Psychology and bestselling author of *Before Happiness* and *The Happiness Advantage*, told me when I interviewed him for his most recent book launch. "Scientifically, happiness is actually a choice we make today and not a state of mind reached in the future. Happiness is also not based on your genes or your external world." According to Shawn, "It's actually not the reality that shapes us, but the lens through which your brain views the world that shapes your reality."

Happiness is *not* the belief that everything is great—happiness is the belief that change is possible. The following are the three greatest predictors of happiness:

- Optimism (the belief your behavior will eventually matter)
- Social connections
- How we perceive stress (as a challenge or as a threat)

I really like Shawn's personal definition of happiness: the joy one feels striving for one's potential, which is exactly what this book is all about. It's about the potential to create life and how we can pursue this potential and enhance our chances to realize this potential. By changing our mindset and our habits, we can actually change the entire trajectory of our lives. And by adapting a spiritual attitude, we may see the grace in our world again and celebrate what we already have, instead of wishing for something else.

One of the most memorable examples of a woman who redefined happiness after having lost five pregnancies is Leah in chapter 4: "I felt that having a baby was the key to my happiness. This was the key to my life; this is what I felt I deserved and I wanted. My happiness was tied to a future child and not to my present." Can you identify with any of these statements? It was her work with Russell Davis that turned things around. He helped her to choose happiness *now* over an elusive dream of a future child. Leah realized how "happy and content I was in my life. I work with children, and I can still feel that love. I still feel blessed with the things I do have, like my health, my partner, all of those things. I have reason to feel grateful and blessed."

Practice Your Happiness

One of the easiest and quickest ways to achieve happiness is a daily gratitude practice. For the next three weeks, focus on all the things in your life that you are grateful for. Each day, write down three things for which you feel gratitude—no repeats, please! You can write them down in your journal or on a piece of paper you can then put into your gratitude jar. Watch it fill up with notes of all the things in your life that bring you joy and happiness. Have your family members contribute to the gratitude jar, too, if they'd like.

Achor recommends that, once a day, you journal about a positive experience you've had within the last twenty-four hours. Another of his suggestions: make the very first email you write one that spreads happiness, by praising or thanking someone you know. This two-minute daily email will make a significant difference in how your day unfolds.

Actively choosing happiness and exercising gratitude on your way to motherhood will also be a tremendously helpful practice once you navigate your new life as a mother. Having one child (or several) brings all of us to the edge of our abilities—and then pushes us over the brink. It's inevitable. It's life. It's messy. It's how we grow. Choose to be happy, especially when you are pushed over the edge, like in the poem I mentioned at the beginning of this pillar. So, come really close to the edge. Closer. Closer. One more step.

And remember: *you will fly.*

Be patient. Honor the present moment. Find joy in the now.

THANK YOU
AND LET'S STAY IN TOUCH

They say it "takes a village to raise a child"—and that's so true—and it also took a township to create *The Joy of Later Motherhood*. When I first envisioned this book, I had no idea the wealth of knowledge, wisdom, and encouragement I would discover through my dozens and dozens of interviews with real-life mature moms and passionate natural fertility experts. I am forever grateful to all the women (and men) who openly and deeply shared their experiences with us in this book. *The Joy of Later Motherhood* would not exist without you!

Thank you to all who contributed open-heartedly and generously to this book and to its message that later motherhood is not only possible but, in fact, perfectly natural.

Now that we know we have a much larger influence over our health and, thus, our fertility—regardless of our age—than we previously realized, I hope we mature women feel less pressured and alone and more optimistic and empowered.

It is also my hope that *The Joy of Later Motherhood* supported you with knowledge you may not have had before, like the connection between your reproductive well-being and your mental and emotional well-being; or that switching your diet to healthy and fertility-increasing foods is another big step toward creating or expanding your family; or that it may be time to make changes in your career as the current stressful position you're in could cost you more than just your sleep.

A book with roughly 250 pages may be all you need on your journey, or it may just scratch the surface for you. Either way, please do make use of the Book

Bonus section I've set up for you at *BettinaGordon.com/Bonus*, which includes additional interviews and articles. This membership area is my thank you to you, my dear reader.

There are many other fascinating topics, especially significant for us older and often accomplished women—like how to achieve the motherhood/C-Suite "balance" or how to increase your energy and vitality as you age—that I write about on my website. If you have big concerns about mature motherhood, please bring them to me as I am more than happy to put my journalistic skills to good use and research and write about the solutions to *your* specific challenge. Pop over to *BettinaGordon.com/Struggles* and drop me a note.

If you already know you'd like more support and would love to go deeper with me, you can reach out to me directly via email at *BettinaBook@bettinagordon. com*. On a limited basis, I personally mentor mature moms-to-be, and I suggest scheduling a twenty-minute exploratory session (again, it's free for you) so we can discuss your needs and wants. I am always happy to hear from women whose paths have crossed with mine, and even if I am not the perfect mentor for you, I may have resources or contacts to people who could be the perfect fit, and I will happily share them with you.

I actually gathered so many nuggets of wisdom and actionable and fun advice that I created a second book called *Sisterhood* (more about it also on my website). The format of this book is like a fireside chat between a curious woman and her older sisters. The younger woman can finally ask all the questions she has around later motherhood, while her older sisters offer the smart and honest answers she craves. *Sisterhood* includes topics like the following:

- Will they call me "grandmother"?
- I am very happy with my husband. Will our relationship suffer if we have a child?
- I am at the height of my career and have enormous responsibilities. How could I find balance between a top job and a child?
- What if something goes wrong? How did you deal with the pain of miscarriages?

- Will I be exhausted beyond belief? Will I regret having waited so long because I am not as fit as I used to be?
- Could I still have a home birth at my age?
- Will I fit in with the other, younger parents? Will people judge me for being an old parent?
- Am I putting an unfair burden on my child, who may need to worry about taking care of elderly parents sooner than his peers?
- As my friends who had children earlier begin to have more freedom, will I feel tied down with my young child?
- And many more questions you may have always wanted to ask…

Choosing motherhood in your late 30s and 40s means that many of your friends may be mothers to teenagers or have even become empty nesters by the time you show up for dinner with them with an infant strapped around your waist. Their experience will be your gain. My beloved Austrian soul-sisters Margot, Michaela, and Doris started their families a decade or two before me and are now my reliable sources for sage advice and humorous reminders, like "No worries, this is just a phase, he'll grow out of it".

I was fortunate enough to create another circle of sisters during my pregnancy. My newly found friendship with Jo, Cindy, Hannah, and Hilary (and later Claudia, Michelle, and Elena) made our first year of new motherhood in our 40s much more fun and less daunting than it could have been otherwise. Together we grew into motherhood without losing ourselves in it. My sisterhood gave me strength and encouragement and offered valuable insights for this book. They are a big reason why I title this book *The Joy of*. . . To all of you awesome ladies, who I love and can always count on, thank you! You ROCK!

Writing this book was no small feat; making it "fit for print" wasn't either. Thank you to Kelly Notaras, founder of KN Literary Arts, and Nikki Van De Car for hooking me up with my champion editor, Rebecca Lotenero. Rebecca, as well as my proofreader, Jennifer Hanchey, had personal interest in *The Joy of Later Motherhood*, which made our collaboration even more exciting. My publisher Morgan James Publishing made the whole production process go smoothly and offered valuable marketing advice that I more than happily accepted. Thank you also to authors Brendon Burchard, Kris Carr, Tony Robbins, Marie Forleo, and my coach and mentor Judymay Murphy, whose work and advice helped me write with enthusiasm and joy. As Judymay says, "The energy you feel writing this book is the energy your readers will feel reading it." Amen.

The biggest burst of gratitude and love I feel is for the two human beings without whom Bettina Gordon-Wayne, mother and author, would not exist: my solid-as-a-rock husband, Joshua, and my mischievous, wild child, Hunter. Because of you, my world is filled with more affection, devotion, laughter, adventure, and gray hair—covered by my professional hairdresser—than I could have ever hoped for!

Xoxo,

Bettina

ABOUT THE AUTHOR

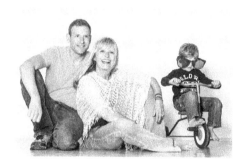

Bettina Gordon-Wayne is an international journalist and certified mental strength trainer with an über-passion for travel. Originally from Vienna, Austria, she has called America home since 1996. At age 44, she became the third generation of women in her family to have healthy children at an age the mainstream deems "dangerous." In *The Joy of Later Motherhood*, Bettina shares the stories and advice of forty women over 40 who all had natural pregnancies and healthy babies to show other women of "advanced maternal age" what is possible and, in fact, perfectly natural. Bettina currently resides in Washington, DC, and Vienna, Austria, with her husband, Joshua, her wild child, Hunter, and Georgia, the squirrel-chasing Pit Bull mix. For more on Bettina's work, visit BettinaGordon.com.

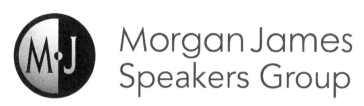

Morgan James
Speakers Group

www.TheMorganJamesSpeakersGroup.com

We connect Morgan James published
authors with live and online events
and audiences who will benefit
from their expertise.

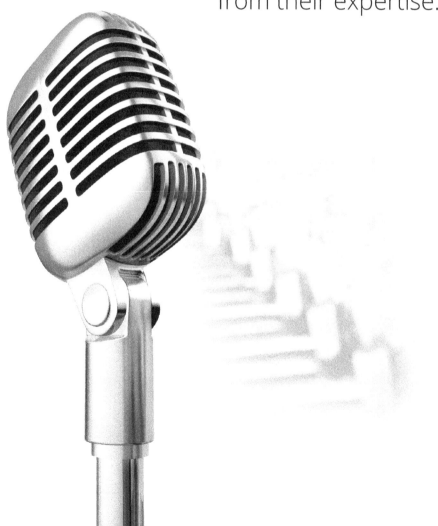